A Child's Eyes

A CHILD'S EYES

A Guide to Pediatric Primary Care

John W. Simon, M.D.

Professor and Chairman, Department of Ophthalmology
Professor of Pediatrics, The Albany Medical College
Albany, New York

Joseph H. Calhoun, M.D.

Director of Pediatric Ophthalmology Services, Wills Eye Hospital
Clinical Professor of Ophthalmology, Thomas Jefferson Medical College
Philadelphia, Pennsylvania

Foreword by Marshall M. Parks, M.D.

Clinical Professor of Ophthalmology
George Washington University School of Medicine
Washington, D.C.

Illustrations by Chris Wikoff

 TRIAD PUBLISHING COMPANY   GAINESVILLE, FLORIDA

Printed in the United States of America

Published and distributed by
Triad Publishing Company
Post Office Box 13355
Gainesville, FL 32604

Library of Congress Cataloging-in-Publication Data

Simon, John W. (John Willard), 1949-.
    A child's eyes : a guide to pediatric primary care / John W.
  Simon, Joseph H. Calhoun ; foreword by Marshall M. Parks ;
  illustrations by Chris Wikoff.
        p.   cm.
    Includes index.
    ISBN 0-937404-52-7 (pbk.)
    1. Pediatric ophthalmology. I. Calhoun, Joseph H.   II. Title.
    [DNLM: 1. Eye Diseases--in infancy & childhood.   2. Eye Diseases-therapy.   3. Diagnostic
Techniques, Ophthalmological--in infancy & childhood.   WW 600 S595c 1998]
RE48.2.C5S55   1998
618. 92'0977--dc21
DNLM/DLC
for Library of Congress   97-48979
                                        CIP

To our own children,
Catherine and Joseph,
Julia and Lia.
And to our young patients —
They make it all worthwhile.

Contents

Foreword

One of the defining characteristics of medical care delivery in the coming era is restriction of access to specialized care. What this means to primary care physicians — to pediatricians and family practitioners—is new responsibility to diagnose and to treat medical problems formerly the province of more specialized physicians. One of the new challenges is that they must decide who should be referred to specialists in pediatric ophthalmology. And increasingly, they must assume the role of educating the parents of their young patients with eye problems.

A Child's Eyes provides a quick desk reference for non-ophthalmological practitioners. It covers the multitude of disorders affecting the eyes of children and gives straightforward descriptions of all the common disorders encountered in pediatric ophthalmology. It is an ideal resource that belongs on the bookshelf of every pediatrician and family practitioner.

The coverage is concise, yet complete, and the book is well illustrated to support the written descriptions. The excellent index and margin references will bring the subject needing review and the practitioner together in an instant.

Eye problems can be difficult for primary care providers, but they can be completely baffling to parents. When a physician is faced with the need to educate parents, *A Child's Eyes* will provide the needed information in layman's English.

Both authors are seasoned educators and renowned pediatric ophthalmologists and strabismologists. They have many years of practice in this field, providing care to untold thousands of children and, in the process, investing enormous time interacting with and educating their parents. Although they have addressed this book principally to primary care physicians, it is designed to be shared with interested parents, as well as with educators, occupational therapists, and the many other professionals concerned with children.

A Child's Eyes is a valuable tool for everyone who is interested in acquiring an understanding of this specialty.

MARSHALL M. PARKS, M.D.

Preface

During the course of our careers as pediatric ophthalmologists, we have encountered countless parents who are genuinely perplexed about their children's eye problems. We wrote this book with the realization that, more and more, it will be primary care practitioners who will have to provide answers to their questions. More importantly, these doctors will also be faced with treating certain patients that they previously referred, and will need the confidence to decide when a patient absolutely requires referral. Insurance administrators and others interested in medical care utilization will want to know this information as well.

We've tried to address this book on two levels: first, for primary care physicians, and second, for parents and other nonmedical professionals who have regular contact with our patients. It's not always been easy. There are doubtless some instances when the text will be too elementary for our medical readers and others when it will be too sophistocated for our lay readers. We trust both will be understanding.

Finally, a note about eye doctors. We're both ophthalmologists, which means we completed medical school, one year of post-graduate training in primary medical care, and three years of residency training in ophthalmology—before subspecializing in pediatric ophthalmology. There are also eye doctors of optometry. They have earned a professional degree (O.D.), in a college of optometry. In general, ophthalmologists do optical treatments (glasses and contact lenses), medical management, and surgery for eye problems. Optometrists spend more of their time on optical treatments, and may specialize in such fields as contact lenses and low vision. The differences in scope of practice between ophthalmology and optometry have narrowed in recent years, causing a certain amount of controversy. We want to side-step this controversy, and so have referred to "eye doctor" in many places, specifying "ophthalmologist" only when the issue is clearly surgical.

John W. Simon, M.D
Joseph H. Calhoun, M.D.

Introduction

*L*ittle Heather was an adorable two-year-old who had her dad—and almost everybody else—wrapped around her little finger. She also had an eye problem.

One day, for no apparent reason, Heather's right eye began to turn inward, or cross. At first Heather's parents weren't sure there really was a problem because her eye crossed only when she was very tired. But gradually the crossing became more pronounced and more frequent. Then it began to happen not only when Heather was tired, but almost all day long. Looking at her picture books made it worse, and she tended to close or cover her right eye.

Her parents began to panic. Her pediatrician referred them to an ophthalmologist, who said that Heather had strabismus. The doctor prescribed a pair of glasses and an eye patch for her left eye. Heather, of course, had no use for either one. Whenever her parents left the room she pulled off the glasses, and the patch came off soon after. Every time, her right eye immediately crossed in again.

Heather's parents were torn. They couldn't stand to see their little girl so uncomfortable. But they were afraid that if they didn't force her to wear the glasses and patch, her vision would be ruined for life. Maybe the doctor had made a mistake. A neighbor said that his son Samuel had once had the same problem as Heather, but a simple operation had corrected it. Surgery sounded awful. But maybe it was better than making Heather do something that made her unhappy and didn't seem to be doing any good.

Heather's story, with minor variations, is repeated every day. Parents are understandably confused and anxious. Eye problems can be complicated, and the technical jargon used to describe them makes them seem even more so. Many parents are afraid that any mistake on their part might damage their children's eyes for the rest of their lives.

It often comes as a surprise to parents that so many different problems can affect how their children see and that so many kinds

Many parents are afraid that any mistake on their part might damage their children's eyes for the rest of their lives.

of treatment may be recommended for problems that, at least at first glance, seem to be identical. When Heather's parents were told that Samuel had had "exactly the same problem" as Heather, the chances are good that the problems weren't really the same at all.

Myths and misconceptions about children's eye problems are widespread. All parents have heard stories about children with "lazy" eyes or "pink" eyes and even such diseases as glaucoma or cataracts. They hear about children who need glasses by age 2 and newborns who need eye surgery. They're convinced that sitting too close to the television or reading with a flashlight under the covers will do permanent damage to their children's eyes.

Parents are surprised to learn:

-- when an eye turns in childhood, its vision may suffer;

-- glasses sometimes make crossed eyes straighten;

-- "vision" is what an eye can see, not what its glasses prescription is;

-- a right eye that is crossed can be straightened by surgery on either eye (or both eyes).

This book will help you answer the questions, explain the unexplained, and dispel the myths and misconceptions about children's eye problems. After reading it you should understand enough about the subject not to panic when something unusual is noticed about a child's eyes or visual behavior. You should know when and where to turn for help and what kinds of tests are likely to be performed. You will be able to answer the questions parents ask in language they can understand.

THE EYE: ANATOMY AND FUNCTION

Before delving into the details of the various problems that can affect children's eyes, we will begin by explaining the parts of the eye itself.

A marvelously adapted organ, the eye is able to give us many times more information about our surroundings than all our other senses combined. Its structure is remarkable, not only for what it can do, but for its inherent beauty as well. Because the eye is the only part of the body where nerves and tiny blood vessels can be seen directly, examining the eye can provide important clues about the health of the entire body.

The eye is often compared to a camera, and the similarities are striking. Just as a camera focuses light on the film, an eye focuses light on the retina. The eye has a variable-focus lens suspended in place just behind the pupil, with more focusing power provided by the curvature of the cornea. Like the aperture of an automatic camera, the pupil opens in dim light and closes in bright light to control the amount of light entering the eye.

Much like the images on a roll of film, images formed on the retina must then be "developed." For this purpose they are transmitted by the optic nerve, which leads from each eye toward the visual area in the back of the brain.

Because the eye is the only part of the body where nerves and tiny blood vessels can be seen directly, examining the eye can provide important clues about the health of the entire body.

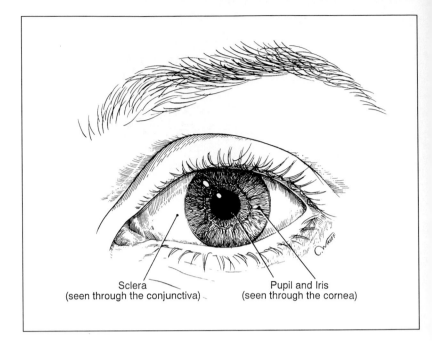

Sclera
(seen through the conjunctiva)

Pupil and Iris
(seen through the cornea)

THE NORMAL EYE. The transparent cornea reflects a small portion of the incoming light, for example from a camera's flash. That reflection is seen as a white spot at the 10:30 o'clock position in front of the iris and pupil.

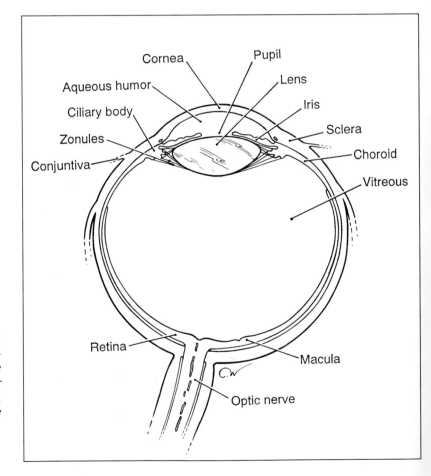

Cornea

Pupil

Aqueous humor

Lens

Ciliary body

Iris

Zonules

Sclera

Conjuntiva

Choroid

Vitreous

Retina

Macula

Optic nerve

THE NORMAL EYE IN CROSS SECTION. The outermost of the three layers includes the transparent cornea and the opaque white sclera. The middle layer is the vascular uvea, made up of the iris, the ciliary body, and the choroid. The innermost layer is the retina.

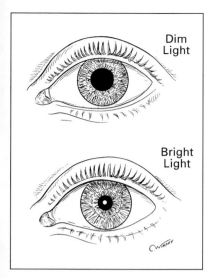

PUPILLARY LIGHT REACTION. Both pupils dilate in dim light and constrict in bright light.

Corneal curvature accounts for about two-thirds of the focusing power of the eye.

The cornea is richly supplied with pain nerves. Infection or damage to the cornea can often threaten eyesight.

How the eye functions

To understand the eye, let's begin by looking at some illustrations of it *(opposite page)*. Note the iris, pupil, conjunctiva, sclera, cornea, choroid, ciliary body, zonules, lens, retina, macula, optic nerve, two kinds of fluid and six muscles. Each of these must be in good working order for the eye to function properly.

The iris and the pupil   Even though it's actually inside the eye, the first part people tend to look at is the *iris* (plural: *irides*). The iris is a muscular structure shaped like a doughnut. Its color is determined by pigment cells, which tend to darken during infancy. Generally by 6 to 12 months of age, the color of the iris is determined for life.

The black hole at the center of the iris is the *pupil.* In darkness it dilates and in light it constricts, due to the involuntary relaxation or contraction of the iris muscles. The pupils also change size in response to looking at things at close range, to different emotional states, and to various kinds of medications and eyedrops.

The sclera and the cornea   The "white" of the eye—the *sclera*—is the tough outer coating that gives the eye its spherical shape (the eyelids conceal much of its shape). During the first few years of life, the sclera is still soft and growing.

The sclera is covered by the *conjunctiva* (plural: *conjunctivae*), a thin membrane, translucent like waxed paper, that also lines the undersides of the eyelids. The conjunctiva, along with the lacrimal glands, makes tears, which keep the eye moist. But it is probably best known for its tendency to get inflamed when it is infected or irritated. This condition, called *conjunctivitis,* is very common and is generally only an annoyance.

The *cornea* is in front of the iris. Though it is part of the same layer as the sclera, it is different in that the cornea is transparent. Light must pass through it to get to the pupil and the inside of the eye. As you can see from the cross section, the cornea is curved like a watchglass. This curvature accounts for about two-thirds of the focusing power of the eye. The cornea is a very sensitive structure. If you have ever had something in your eye, had a scratch on the cornea, or worn a contact lens too long, you are well aware that it is richly supplied with pain nerves. Unlike inflammation or infection of the conjunctiva, damage to the cornea can often threaten eyesight.

The choroid, the ciliary body, and the lens   Hidden beneath the sclera is a second layer, the *choroid.* Its function is to supply blood to the other parts of the eye, especially the retina. In fact, blood vessels in the choroid are more densely packed than anywhere else in the body.

The retina needs a rich supply of blood for two reasons. First, it is metabolically active and therefore needs a great deal of energy. Second, the focusing of light onto the retina creates heat, much like the focusing of the sun's light by a magnifying lens. The rich blood supply of the choroid carries this heat away and protects the eye from injury.

The choroid is in the same layer as the iris. Also in this layer is the *ciliary body*, which lies just behind the junction of the cornea and the sclera. Like the iris, the ciliary body is a muscular structure, but its central opening is much larger. The ciliary body produces *aqueous humor*.

The *lens*, made of nearly pure protein, is a transparent structure with two convex surfaces. Special "guy-wires" called *zonules* connect the lens to the ciliary body and suspend it so it is centered behind the pupil. When the ciliary body constricts, it relaxes the pull on the zonules so that the shape of the lens changes. This process, called *accommodation*, focuses light on the retina so we can see near objects clearly. When the muscles of the ciliary body are relaxed, tension is placed on the zonules and the focus of the lens is readjusted so we can see things at a distance.

Often in older people, and occasionally even in children, the normally transparent lens becomes cloudy. If it interferes with vision, this clouding of the lens is called a *cataract*.

The retina   The innermost layer of the eye is the *retina*, which contains specialized cells called photoreceptors (rods and cones). These cells turn light energy into nerve impulses. In the center of the retina is the *macula* (the very center is called the *fovea*). The central part of the retina provides the sharpest vision because a very large number of photoreceptors are crowded closely together. For that reason, people subconsciously direct their foveas at whatever they're looking at.

The fovea has no blood vessels, but it looks red because of blood that shows through from the choroid. The parts of the retina farther away from the macula are important because they provide us with peripheral vision—a wide visual area around what is directly looked at.

The optic nerve   Nerve impulses from the photoreceptors in all parts of the retina are passed to the *optic nerve*, which can be seen inside the eye as a pinkish-yellow disc.

You can "find" your own optic disc by doing a little experiment. Hold your two forefingers in front of you at arm's length. Now close your left eye, concentrate on the tip of the left finger, and move the right finger slowly to the right. When your fingers are about 6 inches apart, the right fingertip will disappear, only to reappear when the fingers are 7 or so inches apart.

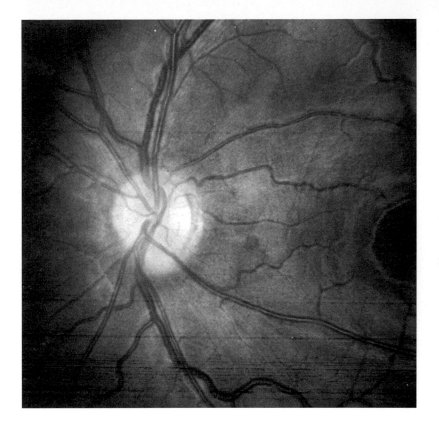

THE NORMAL OPTIC NERVE AND RETINA. Viewed through the indirect ophthalmoscope, the healthy optic nerve appears as a pinkish-yellow disc. The youthful retina reflects light as a sheen, which in this picture nearly encircles the macula, partially seen about two and one-half disc-diameters to the right of the optic nerve.

You've just demonstrated the "blind spot" caused by the optic disc, which contains no photoreceptor cells. It does contain some one million nerve cells, however, which transmit all of the visual information from the eye to the brain. In fact, anatomists consider the optic nerve a part of the brain.

The fluids inside the eye   The front third of the eye—the part behind the cornea and surrounding the lens and iris—is filled with *aqueous humor* (also called *aqueous*). Aqueous is a watery fluid produced by the ciliary body. It circulates through the pupil and filters out of the eye at the angle between the iris and the cornea. The balance between the production and drainage of aqueous maintains the normal pressure inside the eye. If the pressure is too high, usually because of poor drainage, *glaucoma* can develop and the optic nerve can be damaged.

Vitreous humor (also called *vitreous*) fills the back two-thirds of the eye. Vitreous has an unusual consistency, much like uncooked egg white.

Both the aqueous and the vitreous must remain clear for vision to be sharp. Inflammation or blood inside the eye, for example, would likely blur the vision.

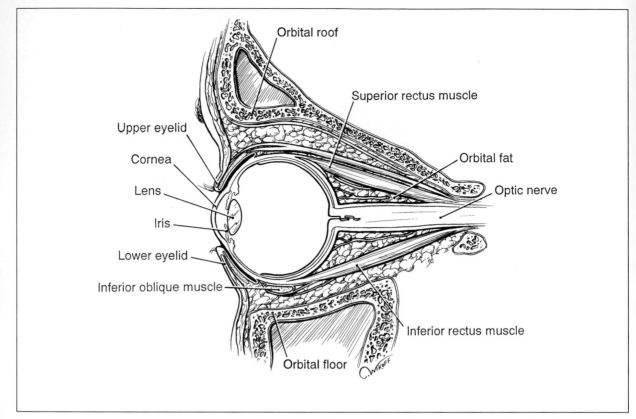

THE NORMAL EYE AND ORBIT IN LONGITUDINAL SECTION. The eye sits in a bony cavity called the orbit (the eye socket). The optic nerve carries visual information to the brain. This view shows the superior rectus and inferior rectus muscles. The medial rectus and lateral rectus muscles are out of the plane of the drawing.

The eyelids and the orbit

In front of the eye, of course, are the eyelids. The lids keep the cornea moist by moving the tears across the surface of the eye with each blink and by preventing the evaporation of tears during sleep. Without normal eyelids, corneal damage often occurs and can be severe.

Tears are made by the *lacrimal glands,* which are located in the outer part of the upper eyelid just beneath the brow. There are also accessory lacrimal glands in the conjunctiva lining the undersides of the lids and covering the sclera.

Eyelids that droop—*ptosis*—are usually not dangerous, though babies with this problem should be checked for amblyopia, or poor vision.

The structures around the eye fill the eye socket, which is called the *orbit.* The eye is protected from injury by the orbital bones and the cushion of fat that surround it. The illustration *(above)* shows how the vital structures of the orbit—the optic nerve, the eye

The lids keep the cornea moist by moving the tears across the surface of the eye with each blink and by preventing the evaporation of tears during sleep.

muscles, and the blood vessels and nerves that supply them—fit neatly together behind the eye.

Farther back in the orbit, the bones tend to be thin and can break easily.

The eye muscles

The six muscles that attach to each eye move the eyes and align them with each other. When they don't work in a coordinated fashion, the result is loss of alignment, or *strabismus*. These muscles are particularly important in pediatric ophthalmology because strabismus usually begins in childhood.

Four of the muscles are oriented straight ahead. They are called the *rectus muscles* from the Latin word for "straight." The other two are called the *oblique muscles* because they pull obliquely.

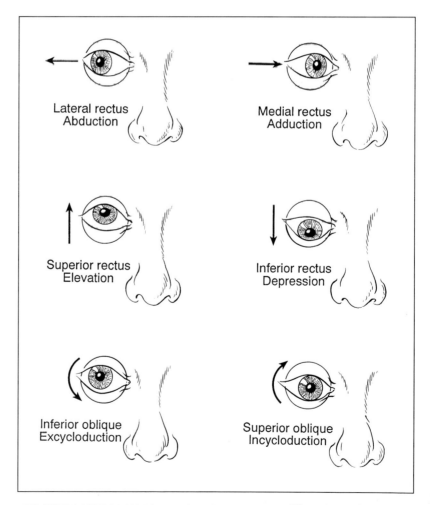

THE EXTRAOCULAR MUSCLES AND THEIR ACTIONS. The principal actions of the six extraocular muscles in the right eye are shown schematically.

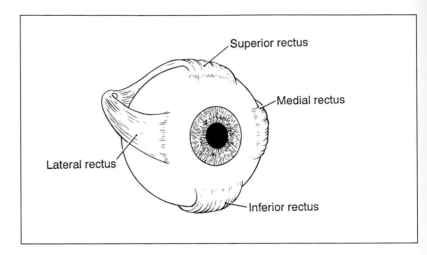

THE RECTUS MUSCLES. This view shows the four rectus muscles of the right eye. The medial and inferior recti are partially hidden behind the eye.

The rectus muscles   The rectus muscles connect to the bones at the back of the orbit. The front end of each muscle attaches to the sclera near the cornea. When these muscles contract, they simply turn the eye (or, more accurately, the cornea) in the direction of their attachments. The *superior rectus* muscle attaches to the sclera above the cornea; when it contracts, the cornea turns up. Similarly, the *inferior rectus* attaches to the sclera below the cornea and turns the cornea down. The *medial rectus* attaches on the inner side and turns the cornea medially (toward the nose), while the *lateral rectus* attaches on the outer side and turns the cornea laterally (away from the nose).

The oblique muscles   The two oblique muscles are a bit more complicated, since they attach near the back of the eye.

Let's look at the *inferior oblique* muscle, which connects the lower half of the back of the eye to the lacrimal bone near the nose. When it contracts, the back of the eye turns down and the front of the eye

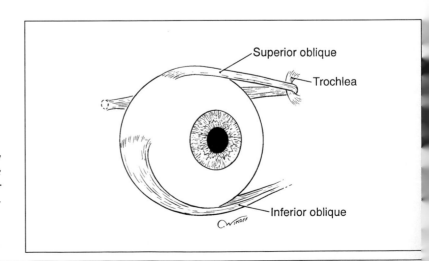

THE OBLIQUE MUSCLES. This view shows the superior and inferior oblique muscles of the right eye. The posterior portion of the superior oblique is partially hidden behind the eye.

turns up. In some children this muscle contracts too much and causes the cornea to turn up too far, especially when it's looking toward the nose. This condition is appropriately called "inferior oblique overaction." The inferior oblique also rotates the eye so that the 12 o'clock position turns away from the nose *(excycloduction)*.

The *superior oblique* muscle attaches to the upper half of the back of the eye, extending backward through the trochlea, a bony pulley near the nose, and finally connecting to the bones at the back of the orbit. When it contracts, the back of the eye rises and the front lowers. This muscle also tends to rotate the eye so that the 12 o'clock position rotates toward the nose *(incycloduction)*. If this muscle is weak, the eye can't turn down well. In fact, this muscle is occasionally weak from birth, and that weakness may cause persistent head tilting.

The path from the optic nerve to the brain

The eye muscles surround the optic nerve as it extends from the eye to the back of the orbit, where it passes through the hole in the skull called the *optic canal*. But before reaching the brain, the optic nerves

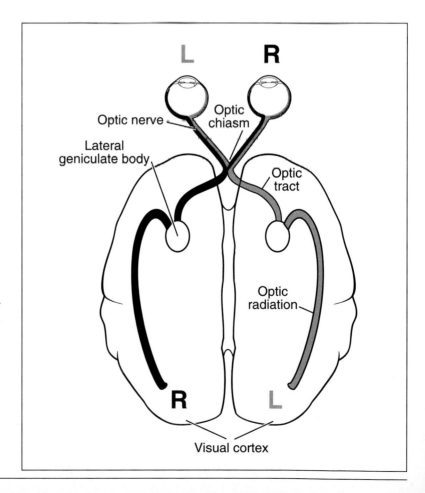

PATHWAY FROM THE EYE TO THE BRAIN. Note that the path from the temporal half of the left eye and the nasal half of the right eye join at the optic chiasm and proceed to the left visual cortex. That pathway, labeled "R" because it images the right visual field in each eye, is shown as a dark line in this drawing.

from both eyes partially cross each other at the *optic chiasm* and form the optic tracts, which end at "relay stations" in the middle of the brain called the *lateral geniculate bodies*. From the lateral geniculate body the optic radiations carry visual information to the occipital cortex. This is the area at the back of the brain that processes the visual information from the photoreceptors in the retina, resulting in visual perception.

Because of the way the optic nerves cross, the right side of the brain allows us to see objects on the left side of our field of vision (imaged in both eyes). Similarly, the left side of the brain allows us to see objects on the right side of our field of vision.

It is a long way from the front of the eye to the back of the brain, and much sensory and motor coordination is needed to keep the process of vision functioning normally. Fortunately, the structures just described work remarkably well together, in most cases without our even having to think about them. For example, parts of the brain subconsciously control the coordinated pull of muscles inside and outside the eyes so that we can shift our gaze in any direction and focus steadily and clearly with our eyes in any position. And the images seen by each eye are integrated by the visual cortex into a single "picture." Considering how complicated vision is and how many ways it might go wrong, it's amazing that most people have so little trouble seeing normally.

EXAMINING THE EYES

1 Early Vision and Early Eye Problems

It is natural for parents to try to establish eye contact with their newborn. That should be possible within the first 4 to 6 months. If it's not, there may be a problem.

Normal visual development

At first, a newborn baby's eyes are closed most of the day, and both attention span and control of eye movements are poorly developed. When they do begin to use their eyes, babies are more interested in things that are close to them than in things that are far away. They are easily capable of seeing across the room, but they find something closer to them more interesting. Of course, even normal newborns may not respond consistently.

Just as they develop in other ways, young children develop *visual acuity* as they get older. Visual acuity is a measurement of the ability to see. It will be discussed in detail later. For now, it's enough to know that 20/20 is normal, 20/40 is good enough to drive a car, and 20/200 (the size of the "big E" on the eye chart) is considered to be legally blind.

Visual acuity is a measurement of the ability to see.

Newborn babies normally have visual acuity good enough to see a face across a room. By the time they reach their first birthday, their acuity has improved to 20/100 or so. By the second birthday, they have 20/30 vision. By the third birthday, some children can see 20/20. Naturally, there is considerable normal variation at all these ages.

When should children begin routine eye exams?

A child's eyes and visual function can be evaluated at any age, even in the newborn nursery. But unless there are symptoms suggesting an eye problem or there is a family history of concern to the family or the primary care physician, most children do not require an examination by an eye doctor. We believe that "routine exams" by eye doctors are not needed unless there is some problem or condition that is suspected or needs to be followed up on.

Most children do not require an examination by an eye doctor.

But *screenings* by primary care physicians should be performed routinely, beginning in the newborn period. As soon as a child can name the pictures on an eye chart, it's important to measure visual acuity. (Visual function is much easier to test after about 6 months of age, and visual acuity can be measured beginning about age 3.) Most children have their vision tested yearly at school.

Parents should be aware of certain symptoms that may be warning signs of eye problems and may require consultation with an eye doctor. Some of these are

○ rubbing the eyes excessively
○ continually closing one eye
○ tearing or unusual light sensitivity
○ red, itchy or swollen eyes
○ not being able to see something others can see
○ eyestrain when reading
○ an eye that crosses or wanders

Impaired vision

A slight vision impairment may escape detection for a long time, possibly even until a child is about kindergarten age. Most toys are large and young children hold them quite close. Especially in familiar surroundings, preschool children with poor vision may function very well. On the other hand, watching television at close range does not necessarily mean there's a problem. Almost all children sit close to the television.

Over time, the world that's of interest to a child moves farther away and, especially when the child is introduced to blackboard work at school, even mild problems become apparent. Children with mild-to-moderate visual impairments often begin to have trouble in elementary school. It's not that their vision has become worse; rather the demands on their vision have changed. For the first time they have to see finer print and smaller distant objects.

When a visual impairment is severe, the child's eyes may be in constant motion (called *nystagmus*). Some children may simply be unable to direct their gaze (*fixate*) at all. If visual impairment of any degree is found or even suspected, an ophthalmologist should be consulted.

Excessive tearing and associated problems

The tear ducts, which drain tears from the eyes to the nose, should open before the first birthday.

Tearing in infancy is so common a problem that many specialists consider it normal during the first few months. The tear ducts, which drain tears from the eyes to the nose, should open before the first birthday; when they do, the problem goes away. Many ophthalmologists and primary care physicians recommend intermittent antibiotic eyedrops or ointment, and massage of the tear sac (more about this later). If the discharge does not clear after the first year, or if it is very bad even earlier, a surgical probing may be recommended to open the tear ducts.

Sometimes, in addition to tearing, the child is sensitive to light or has what looks like a pink or red eye. These symptoms may be associated with more serious problems, such as inflammation inside the eye (*uveitis* or *iritis*), irritation of the cornea, or glaucoma. (In infants, glaucoma also makes the eye grow too large and the cornea turn cloudy.) Therefore, if tearing is associated with light sensitivity, pink eye, enlargement or clouding of the cornea, or poor visual behavior, the child should be evaluated promptly by an ophthalmologist.

Tearing associated with light sensitivity or pink eye may be associated with serious eye problems.

Strabismus and amblyopia

The vision problem that commonly accompanies strabismus is called *amblyopia.* It is frequently referred to as "lazy eye." Some people use the term lazy eye to mean strabismus, but that isn't quite correct; lazy eye means loss of vision from amblyopia. Strabismic amblyopia can usually be cured if it is recognized and treated during early childhood.

Most children whose eyes turn have few other symptoms. But some—especially those who are toddler age and older—may also experience visual discomfort when the eye first turns. Children of this age may not be able to verbalize their discomfort, but the telltale signs are closing or covering one eye, complaining of double vision, or holding the head in a peculiar position.

Telltale signs of strabismus include closing or covering one eye, double vision, or holding the head in a peculiar position.

Occasionally, eyes with strabismus have more serious structural problems. Examples include cataract, glaucoma, and damage to the retina or optic nerve.

Less common problems

Parents may notice that their child's pupil is not uniformly black (or, in photographs, uniformly red). This observation may mean that some abnormality is blocking the clarity of the eye. Although a cataract is what you would logically think of first in this situation, such a blockage may be anywhere from the cornea, in the front of the eye, to the retina in the back. More serious causes, such as retinal detachment or tumor, are rare.

❦

All of the problems mentioned in this chapter are covered in more detail later. But first we need to discuss how children's eyes are examined—whether by eye doctors or by primary care physicians.

2   How Children's Eyes Are Examined

The attention span of young children is so limited that the eye examination usually begins as soon as the doctor enters the examining room. Simple observations can give important clues to a multitude of disorders. Roving eye movements and visual inattention, for example, may signify severe visual impairment. Light sensitivity may suggest corneal irritation, glaucoma or inflammation inside the eye. An abnormally small cornea may herald an optic nerve abnormality. Until the age of 5 or so, each child must be allowed to set the limits, or at least the order, of what is done.

Examining the eyes of a school-age child is usually a pleasure —for both the doctor and the patient. After about age 4, children want to participate, and their responses are quick and accurate. It's the little ones who present the real challenge. Toddlers have learned that doctors do things that hurt, and they would really rather be somewhere else, thank you. Babies are likely to be just as frightened, but they may also simply ignore the doctor and anything having to do with the examination.

Occasionally parents will ask, "Why didn't Dr. So-and-So tell us about this problem two years ago?" It may be that it hadn't developed yet, but it may also have been too hard to detect when the child was younger. It's a good idea, if you still think there's a problem that one examination did not reveal, to re-evaluate or get a consultation.

The first two years

Children's eyes can be examined as early as the first few days of life. But the examination may not be easy. Of course, the doctor expects little cooperation at this stage and feels lucky if the child's eyes are even open. Often the lids will open widely when the room lights are first dimmed. This response, called "eye popping," gives evidence of at least some visual function. Even in very young babies the pupils react to a change in light unless an abnormality is present.

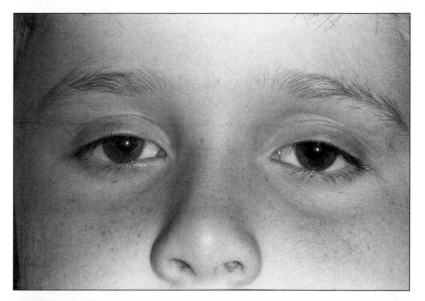

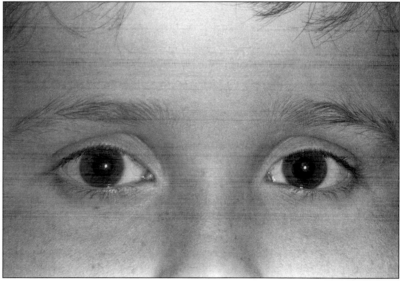

THE EYE POPPING REFLEX. Infants normally open their eyes widely and occasionally look downward when the room lights are first dimmed. The upper picture was taken with the room lights on; note the constricted pupils. The lower picture was taken when the room lights were dimmed; note the dilated pupils.

Children from 3 months to 2 years or so like to play peek-a-boo. If they will look at a face or at a small toy using the right eye, for example, they should do the same with the left. If they can't, or if they push away the card or the hand used to cover the right eye, the vision in the left eye may be poor.

Some children in this age range will reach for small objects that are held in front of them. One strategy is to use those colorful little candy sprinkles that bakeries put on cupcakes. Because they're sweet, a child will sometimes even let the doctor put a piece of tape over one eye, and then over the other, to test each eye separately. It can be dramatic to see a child who has eagerly seized and eaten the candy when one eye was tested begin to grope for the candy when that eye is covered and the other is tested. After the first birthday, these tricks work more and more reliably. Moving small objects farther away can uncover more subtle vision problems.

Meeting the challenges presented by a frightened and unco-operative child is essential for the examination to be fruitful, perhaps more in our field than in any other pediatric subspecialty. After all, the pediatric cardiologist may be able to hear a few heart sounds during the brief seconds between screams. But crying babies will let the eye doctor know very little about their vision—except, of course, that they can see a fearsome object the size of a person wearing a white coat. There are many successful strategies, but they must fit both the personality of the doctor and the needs of each individual child.

Ages two to four

About the time of the second birthday, children can become willing participants in the examination. They have to be coaxed, of course, and sometimes eye doctors spend a lot of effort convincing children they don't intend to hurt them. The goal, in fact, is to make them think that they are about to play a game that's lots of fun.

A good beginning is "slapping five," a nearly universal greeting from about the age of 2. At some level this seems to establish a relationship of trust between child and doctor. The next step is to coax the child into an automatic chair, either alone or on a parent's lap. Children may be asked to "test their arm muscles" by lifting up on the arms of the chair while the doctor pushes the pedal that raises it.

The instruments used for the examination become "toys," and the doctor needs an assortment (it is often said that "one toy is good for one look"). Long attention spans are not characteristic of 2- and 3-year-olds, and it's important to move quickly using a variety of stimuli. One of the most useful toys is the penlight, which can reveal many abnormalities that may affect vision. A common strategy is to ask the child to "blow out the light" while quickly using it to check the pupils and the front part of the eyes for obvious abnormalities that can signal specific problems.

Although most toys are held close to the child, some mechanical toys and perhaps a television set may be at the end of the room, electronically controlled by foot pedals. For example, a bear might beat a drum to applaud the child who correctly names the pictures on an eye chart. Or a video movie may come on when the child's "magic nose" is twisted, and turn off when the child's "magic ear" is pulled. Because they think they're controlling these stimuli themselves, children seem more attracted to them.

Dilating the pupils

Dilating the pupils is important because an adequate examination may simply not be possible otherwise. Through the widely dilated pupil, abnormalities can be seen inside the eye that might be hidden behind an undilated iris. Just as important, the eye drops that dilate the pupil (mydriatics) also relax the muscles of the ciliary body (i.e., they are also cycloplegics) so that glasses can be more accurately prescribed if they're needed. Otherwise, spontaneous changes in the child's focus would make the prescription difficult to determine.

We're sometimes asked whether primary care physicians should use drops to dilate the pupils for screening examinations. The answer is, on an occasional basis, *yes* (one drop of tropicamide 1% in each eye). In some cases, drops may save an unnecessary referral—for example, because the red reflex is dimmed by a darkly pigmented eye. Certainly, primary care physicians are equipped to deal with the rare side effects, including fever, flushing, and tachycardia. But it is not currently standard care to use the drops in this way. (An ophthalmologist will almost certainly use a cycloplegic drop as part of the initial examination.)

Getting the eyedrops into the eye can be a challenge. A favorite trick is to tell children the drops "tickle" and they'll have to wipe them out with a tissue "right away" or they'll start to laugh. This trick works about two-thirds of the time. At least the child usually smiles. Some doctors use an anesthetic drop first, so the sting is mild and goes away while they child is still distracted by the wiping.

CHARACTERISTICS AND DOSAGES OF CYCLOPLEGIC AGENTS

CYLCLOPEDIC AGENT	CONCEN- TRATION	USUAL AGE RANGE	DOSAGE	CYCLOPLEGIC EFFECT*	AVG. DURATION OF MAXIMUM MYDRIASIS	CYCLOPLEGIA
Atropine sulfate (sol. or oint.)	1/4% 1/2% 1%	Under 1 1-3 2-10	1 drop t.i.d.	1-2 days for 3 days	10–12 days	12-18 days
Scopolamine (sol. or oint.)	1/4%	3-10	2 drops	30–60 min.	2–3 days	3–4 days
Homatropine hydrobromide	2% 5%	5-20 5-20	5 drops 2 drops	45–60 min.	24–36 hrs.	24–36 hrs.
Cyclopentolate (Cyclogyl)	1/2% 1% 2%	25+ 10-35 5-20	2 drops	20–45 min.	18–24 hrs.	18–24 hrs.
Cyclopentolate + phenylephrine (Cyclomydril)	1%	30+	1 or 2 drops	20–45 min.	18–24 hrs.	18–24 hrs.
Tropicamide (Mydriacil)	1% 2%	25+ 15+**	2 drops	15–20 min.	4–6 hrs.	4–10 hrs.

*Mydriasis begins earlier than cycloplegia in each instance.

**Used alone, tropicamide is a *variable* cycloplegic agent; hence, measurement of residual accommodation is mandatory following its use.

Excerpted from *The Fine Art of Prescribing Glasses without Making a Spectacle of Yourself* by Milder & Rubin. © 1991 Triad Publishing Co.

The fearful child

Sometimes it's hard to avoid tears, but crying rarely means the child is hurting. Fear is the problem. The best techniques may not help the child to be less fearful, but they do manage to get the exam accomplished with minimal discomfort.

For example, if glaucoma is suspected the eye pressure may have to be measured. To get an accurate measurement, the child may have to be held down for a minute or so with the child's head on a parent's knees. The same position works well for children who may simply need to have their lids held open for routine examination of the retina or for examination following an injury.

Often various parts of the eye will need to be examined in great detail. A slit lamp, which directs a slit of light and greatly magnifies the eye, may be used to examine the front part of the eye. The child's chin must be placed on a chin rest and the forehead pressed against a strap. When this examination is essential, it can be performed with the help of one or two adults to hold the child's head in place.

Similarly, specialized techniques such as ultrasonography, to study parts of the eye behind a cataract, or electroretinography, to look for retinal disorders, can be performed with minimal discomfort.

Some children become unconsolably frightened. When this happens while putting drops into the eyes or at any other point, it's best to restrain the child, gently but firmly, and get the unpleasantness over as fast as possible. Trying to reason with a terrified 3-year-old is rarely productive, and it's amazing how quickly they forget once the experience is over.

If a particular examination is essential but cannot be performed otherwise, the doctor may have to use a restraining board, prescribe sedation, or schedule an examination under anesthesia.

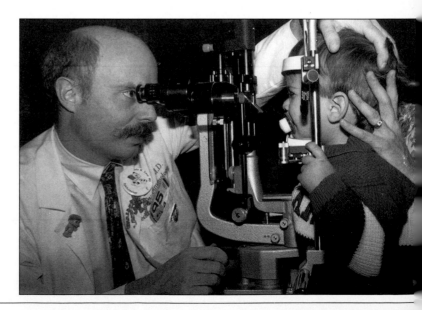

SLIT LAMP EXAMINATION. The slit lamp, which greatly magnifies the eye, can be used to examine young children with the assistance of one or more adults.

3

How Vision Is Tested

The father of one of our young patients telephoned, furious because he had just learned, after a school screening test, that his son was "legally blind" and no one had ever told him. In reality, the child's corrected visual acuity was 20/20; he just didn't happen to have his glasses the day the test was done.

❧

It's ironic, but the most fundamental part of the eye examination is one of the most misunderstood. Most people think of their vision as how they see without their glasses. But eye doctors think of vision as *corrected visual acuity*. This is a measure of the smallest object an eye can see with glasses or contact lenses, if needed.

The best corrected visual acuity is the most important single assessment of the health of an eye.

Indeed, the best corrected visual acuity is the most important single assessment of the health of an eye, and of the entire visual system. In most cases, there is no reason even to measure uncorrected acuity.

Eye doctors devote so much effort to measuring corrected visual acuity because our first goal is to improve it.

The glasses prescription

Children who wear glasses generally see normally when the glasses are on. So it's natural for parents to think that thick glasses are equivalent to poor vision. They frequently hope that the effect of correction will be therapeutic so that in time the glasses will no longer be needed. "Will my child's vision get better?" really means "Will the prescription gradually get weaker or be less needed?"

Unfortunately, there are two facts that are often misunderstood, and the result is too often a thoroughly confused parent.

The strength of the prescription needed is genetically deter-

Eyes that are nearsighted will usually get more nearsighted during the school years and eyes that are farsighted tend to get less farsighted -- no matter what we do about the glasses.

We usually speak of the visual acuity of each eye separately, since a child may see well with one eye and not the other.

mined. Whether we wear our glasses (or contact lenses) or not, and whether they have been made accurately or not, will not alter the prescription that we need to have. To be sure, infants or toddlers who don't receive a needed prescription may suffer a loss of best-corrected visual acuity from amblyopia. And children who don't wear the glasses they need for farsightedness may have trouble accepting the full prescription later. But eyes that are nearsighted will usually get more nearsighted during the school-age years and eyes that are farsighted tend to get less farsighted—no matter what we do about the glasses.

Many children do not see normally with both eyes, especially before medical or surgical treatment . . . no matter what glasses are used. We remember one unfortunate child who went blind from a tumor that destroyed both of his optic nerves. His parents were convinced that if only we'd prescribe glasses, he'd be able to see again. Fortunately, with medical treatment, including an eye patch or surgery as well as glasses, considerable improvement in vision can usually be achieved (depending on the problem, of course).

How vision is tested

Tests of visual acuity measure the smallest object that each eye can see at a certain distance. For verbal children, a test chart is projected across the room, and their responses allow the doctor to measure the child's vision. The vision of each eye is usually tested separately. Children can be very clever "peeking" with their better eye, so we must be particularly careful to make sure that each eye is really tested separately. Sometimes an opaque occluder can be taped over one eye while the other eye is being tested.

TESTING ONE EYE AT A TIME. Placing a piece of opaque tape over the opposite eye assures that the child cannot peak. In this way, poor vision in one eye can be detected.

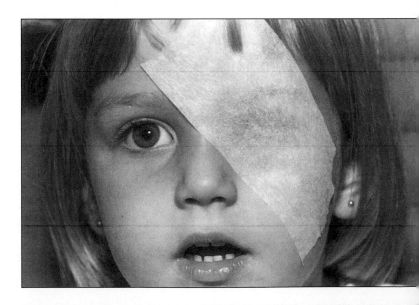

Almost all tests of vision depend on the child's active participation. As a result, children who have a normal visual system but a developmental impairment may test poorly. Three-year-old Tommy, who has trouble paying attention, and 4-year-old Susan, who cannot easily name the pictures in the test, might give up prematurely even though they could readily see the smaller pictures.

Children with more serious developmental impairments may also have visual system involvement. If, for example, parts of the brain that process visual information are abnormal, poor test results will not be a matter of poor attention or communication. The images are lost in processing.

Other children can process the images, but have trouble reacting to them. Richard may be directed to squeeze his lids together in response to a bright light. If there is no response, we might wrongly assume that he can't see the light, when in fact the trouble may be that he doesn't understand the instructions or perhaps isn't able to squeeze his lids.

Children whose eyes are normal and who seem to see poorly because of developmental problems affecting the brain sometimes become more visually responsive over time.

Tests of visual acuity

Many different tests of visual acuity have been developed over the years. The one used for adults and older children is almost always the Snellen eye chart. Children who can't read an eye chart may be tested with pictures or other symbols. Some of the tests used to "measure" the vision of very young children are indirect.

The Snellen eye chart   More than one hundred years ago, a Dutch ophthalmologist named Hermann Snellen invented the eye chart that is named after him. The chart has letters or numbers that are presented at a specified distance.

In general, the specified testing distance is 20 feet. Therefore the top number in the familiar visual acuity fraction is almost always 20. The bottom number in the fraction refers to a "normal" eye.

Let's look at some examples. By definition, normal visual acuity is 20/20. But suppose we're measuring the vision of an eye that sees only half as well as normal. At 20 feet (the top number), it sees what the normal eye sees at 40 feet (the bottom number). So, this particular eye sees 20/40. An eye that sees only one-tenth as well as normal sees 20/200 and is considered legally blind. Some eyes see even better than normal, say 20/15. A person with 20/15 vision can see at 20 feet a letter on the eye chart that is so small that a "normal" person would have to bring it to 15 feet in order to see.

VISION CHARTS. Two of many types that can be hung from a wall or the back of an examining room door. The chart at tleft shows the classical Snellen letters. The one to the right has been adapted for preschool children.The equivalent 20/40 line shows the star, the moon, the circle, and the flag.

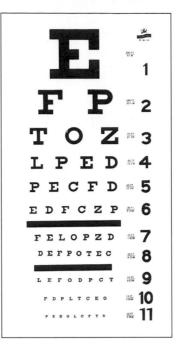

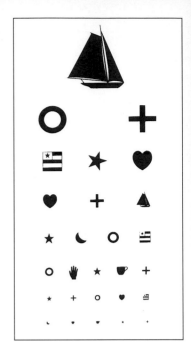

Tumbling E, HOTV, and Allen pictures   Some children who do not know their letters well can be taught the Tumbling E game, in which they simply point in the direction that the "fingers" of the test E are pointing. Children younger than about age 4 seem to have trouble with this task, so the HOTV system may be used instead. One of these letters is projected on a wall and the child points to the same letter on a card.

Allen pictures are another option for young children. Six familiar shapes are projected. The drawbacks here are that some of the

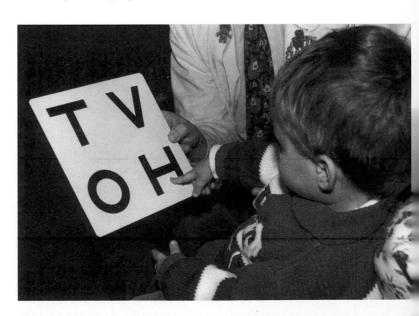

THE HOTV TEST. The child points to the shape (really one of four letters) which matches the letter he sees presented on the vision chart across the room.

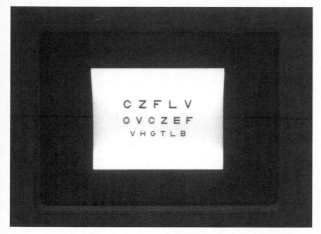 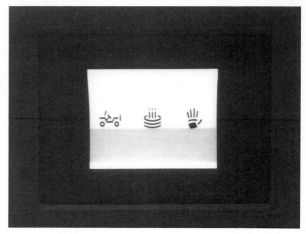

VIDEO-BASED VISION CHARTS. The B-VAT ® system presents various figures appropriate for preschool or older children. One advantage is that it can show pictures (Allen pictures) smaller than conventional projected charts.

shapes are much easier to recognize than they should be, and in most charts the pictures get no smaller than those a child with 20/30 vision can see. The video-based B-VAT® system can present smaller figures equivalent to 20/20.

Whichever test is used, young children may do better when they learn the test at arm's length before it's given from across the room. The visual acuity should not be measured at arm's length, though; such testing is too easy and the results too variable. Similarly, tests using single symbols or letters are easier and give more variable results than those using a series (often called a "line"), but these are sometimes the only choice for young children who need to have a simple test to hold their interest.

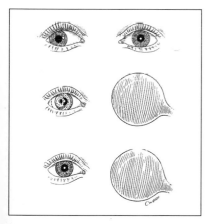

THE COVER TEST. Because children who have strabismus almost always use their better eye, even small angle strabismus in one eye (top) often indicates poor vision in the eye that turns. In this illustration, the right eye centers when the left eye is covered (center). We suspect that the right eye does not see as well as the left eye, especially if the right eye drifts again when the cover is removed (bottom).

Tests for younger children For children who are too young for their vision to be tested using any eye chart, the most commonly used test of vision is somewhat primitive. We first get the child's attention with some object, such as a light, a face, or a small toy. Then we move the object and note whether and how well the child's eyes follow the movement. Ideally the object should be small and far away, but it must be large enough to attract the child's attention.

Children with poor vision in one eye may not be able to direct their gaze (*fixate*) or to follow as well with the bad eye. When the good eye is covered, they may object or simply lose interest. If they can fixate with the bad eye, and if that eye is turned (*strabismic*), as it often is, it will move to center when the good eye is covered. This "cover test" can be a sensitive test of how well one eye sees compared to the other. Children (and adults) who have strabismus almost always use their better eye.

The problem with this kind of testing, of course, is that it is not

Children (and adults) who have strabismus almost always use their better eye.

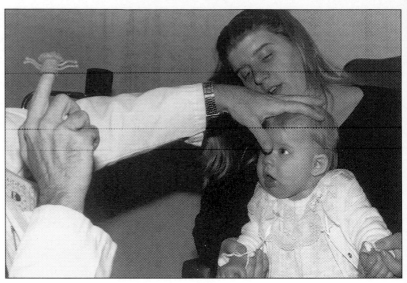

ASSESSING VISION IN A PREVERBAL CHILD. A normal child will be equally happy looking at the toy with either eye covered.

quantitative. It doesn't tell us, in numbers, how well one child—or one eye—sees compared to "normal" or even to last month's measurement.

Quantitative vision tests for preverbal children   There are three kinds of tests that can quantitatively measure the visual acuity of preverbal children. In each case a pattern is presented repetitively and the response is measured; the pattern becomes smaller until the child can no longer respond. The smallest pattern that elicits a response is a measure of the child's visual acuity.

○   One test is based on *optokinetic nystagmus*, a normal involuntary reflex. If a pattern of vertical stripes is passed horizontally across the field of vision, the eyes will follow one stripe for a while and then jerk back to follow another stripe. To use this reflex to test visual acuity, the examiner watches the child's eyes move as the stripes become smaller and smaller, until the jerking of the eyes stops, indicating that the child can no longer distinguish the stripes. This test is rarely used clinically.

○   The *preferential looking test* also depends on reflex behavior and is based on the fact that young children prefer to look at striped patterns rather than blanks. The most often used version is the *Teller acuity card system*. The child is shown stripes of various sizes, sometimes on the left side and sometimes on the right. In each trial there is a blank on the side opposite the stripes. The examiner watches the child's head and eye movements. When the stripes are so small they can no longer be seen, the child stops looking at them.

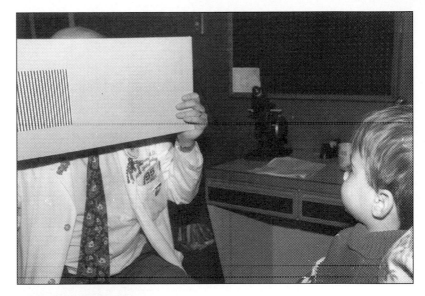

TELLER ACUITY CARDS. The stripes are more interesting than the plain gray portion of the card. Through a peephole in the center of the card, the observer watches the child's responses as different sized stripes are shown to the left or right.

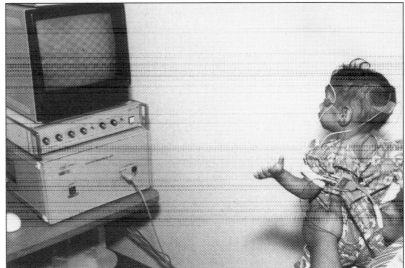

VISUAL EVOKED RESPONSE. Brain waves are recorded from the visual cortex by electrodes taped to the child's scalp as she looks at a variable pattern on the TV screen.

○   The third test doesn't require the child to do anything but look at a pattern on a TV screen. Wires are taped to the child's scalp to record the brain waves evoked by the pattern as it is shown repetitively. The response, aptly named the *visual evoked response*, disappears when the pattern is made so small that it cannot be seen. This test is useful for children who are unable to follow patterns or to redirect their gaze because of developmental problems.

Testing the field of vision

Visual acuity has to do with how well we can see what we're looking at. But it's also important for us to see what may be coming from the side *(peripheral vision)* and to find the thing we want to look at.

Peripheral vision is measured in cooperative adults with a computerized visual field test. Young children, however, cannot perform a formal visual field test, which would require them to concentrate on a single point and push a button when they see a small light appear to one side. But children can have disorders of the eye or the visual parts of the brain that do affect the visual field. So doctors may try to assess the field of vision by bringing a toy around the side of a child's head, looking for eye movement to show that that field is intact.

Testing color vision

About one of every 17 boys has trouble distinguishing shades of red and green (girls are rarely affected). Color blindness is not a very important functional problem in most cases, but it can be a nuisance when trying to match socks or use color-coded educational materials. It hardly ever explains a 3-year-old's difficulty in learning colors. Children who are old enough are asked to name shapes or numbers printed in a mosaic of colored dots that are designed to be hard for color blind people to see. Actually, color "blindness" is almost always an inaccurate term, since most people with color deficiency can see bright colors just fine.

Color deficiency is discussed in more detail in Chapter 18. We now turn our attention to the more common problem of refractive errors and their correction.

4 Why Some Children Need Glasses

Jamie's mother objected when the eye doctor said that her ten-year-old daughter needed glasses for school. "I started wearing glasses when I was in the third grade, just for board work," she lamented. "By the time I was in the seventh grade I was wearing them all the time, and I've worn them every day since. The same thing happened to my older brother and to his middle son. I'm afraid Jamie will get dependent on glasses if she starts wearing them so young.

"How do I know Jamie really needs glasses?"
"Can she get contact lenses instead?"
"Will her eyes get worse?"
"How about eye exercises? "

Two houses down the street from Jamie lives Billy. By general agreement, he is the cutest 3-year-old on the block. Not only does he have short blond hair and an infectious manner; he also has beautiful blue eyes that are emphasized by his glasses, which make his eyes look even bigger and brighter.

At the local swimming pool, Jamie's mother has noticed that one of Billy's eyes turns in toward his nose whenever he takes off his glasses to jump in the deep end with his father. When he splashes in the baby pool, laughing nearly constantly, he would rather wear wet glasses than take them off.

Billy's cousin Ruth has worn glasses for astigmatism since kindergarten. In fact, nearly everyone in the family has astigmatism. They all see well, at least with their glasses on, and none of them seems to know exactly what is wrong with their eyes.

How the eyes process light

To explain the conditions that cause people to need glasses, we must start with some information about elementary optics—the study of light and its relation to seeing.

Rays of light originate from a variety of sources: the sun, light bulbs, a fire, and so on, and they travel through space until they hit something. If that something is opaque, like a flower or tree, the light is either absorbed or reflected. The color of the light that is reflected determines the color we see.

Refraction is the bending of light as it passes from one transparent substance to another.

However, if the light rays hit something transparent, such as air or water or glass or the cornea of the eye, the light passes through it and the path of the light rays is bent, or refracted. *Refraction* is the bending of light as it passes from one transparent substance to another.

In the normal eye of a person looking at a flower, the multitude of light rays reflected by the flower are bent by the cornea and lens so that they come to a single point, the *focal point*, on the retina. The light rays then initiate an extremely complex process in the retina that leads to the visual image in the mind of the viewer.

A defect in refraction is called a refractive error, which means "blurred vision that can be corrected with glasses."

If the image is out-of-focus—that is, if it is not clear in our mind—there is probably something wrong with the way the light was bent (refracted). This defect in refraction is called a *refractive error.* Eye doctors use the words refractive error as an all-encompassing term for "blurred vision that can be corrected with glasses."

There are three basic categories of refractive errors: *myopia* (nearsightedness), *hyperopia* (farsightedness), and *astigmatism.* Presbyopia is another optical cause of blurred vision.

Myopia (nearsightedness)

Jamie, her mother, her mother's brother, and his middle son all have myopia.

Jamie's mother's concerns are typical of those many parents have when they are told that their child could benefit from glasses. This mother's own history of wearing glasses occasionally as a child, needing them more and more during her school years, and then wearing them constantly as an adult is also typical of the majority of people who wear glasses. Those people have the refractive error called *myopia*—they are nearsighted.

Myopes (people with myopia) can best see objects that are close to their eyes; things that are far away are blurred.

Near objects are naturally in focus for the myopic eye; hence the term nearsighted.

If we could peek into a nearsighted eye from the side, we would see that the light rays reflected from an object at close range come to a focal point on the retina, which makes this object easily seen in sharp focus. On the other hand, light rays reflected from a faraway object enter the eye and converge *before* reaching the retina. As a result, this object will be out-of-focus.

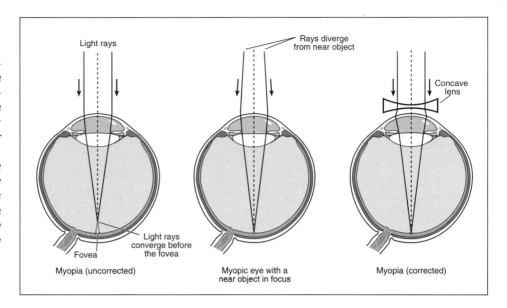

THE OPTICS OF MYOPIA. Left: Light rays from far-away objects come to a focus in front of the retina (fovea), causing a blurred image. Center: Light rays from a near object, on the other hand, are clearly focused on the retina. Right: A concave lens bends the light rays from a distant object in such a manner that they are clearly focused on the retina.

Glasses for myopia　Glasses with lenses that are thinner in the center than on the edges (concave) can optically compensate for myopia—can correct it—by bringing the light rays from a distant object to a focus on the retina. Like glasses for refractive errors of all sorts, they do not eliminate the cause of the refractive error; clear vision is restored only when the glasses are worn.

As with glasses for refractive errors of all sorts . . . clear vision is restored only when the glasses are worn.

When myopia starts　Nearly all myopia begins between ages 6 and 16. It starts at that time with such frequency that it is appropriately called "school-age myopia." Prior to its onset, the eyes were optically normal; they saw clearly with 20/20 vision.

In the normal course of events, myopia tends to be detected reasonably early through annual vision screenings at school or in the office of the pediatrician or family doctor. Sometimes children complain to their parents that they have trouble seeing the blackboard at school.

A common sign of myopia is squinting, squeezing the lids nearly closed in order to see better. Many myopes do this when they are not wearing their glasses, subconsciously taking advantage of a simple optical principle called the "pinhole effect." Viewing things through a small opening like a pinhole, or nearly closed lids, makes out-of-focus images a bit clearer whenever a refractive error blurs them.

A few children become myopic very early in life, within the first several years. The parents usually notice that these children get very close to things they are interested in. Myopia that starts in infancy is often more severe than school-age myopia, but it tends to remain relatively stable over time.

What the myopic child can see When the blurring first becomes symptomatic, most cases of myopia are fairly mild, perhaps around 20/60. Small objects are blurred when they are farther away than 10 feet or so. When glasses are given the child wears them as needed, for blackboard work and perhaps at the movies. At home, things are closer and therefore clearer, and there is no visual gain from wearing the glasses.

Jamie's mother is concerned that by the time her daughter becomes an adult, she will probably wear glasses (or contact lenses) all the time. Unfortunately for Jamie and for millions of others like her, school-age myopia is progressive, generally until the body stops growing. The distance beyond which things begin to blur, the far-point of clear vision, gradually becomes closer and closer. To maintain clear vision, Jamie's glasses will need to be made stronger as the myopia increases—typically once or twice a year.

There is a second factor in the gradual increase of wearing time. As children get older, they need clearer vision to see the increasing amount of detail in their ever-expanding world. Fifteen-year-old boys hit baseballs 200 feet instead of the 50 feet a child hits a T-ball. In school, teachers introduce algebra and exponents, write more and smaller letters on the blackboard, and so on. Even if their myopia does not increase, older children find more situations in which the clear vision they can have with their glasses is advantageous.

Hyperopia (farsightedness)

In childhood, the hyperopic eye generally sees near and far objects equally well; the term farsighted does not mean that children see objects in the distance more clearly.

Billy, the 3-year-old whose glasses make his eyes look bigger, has hyperopia. The popular name, farsightedness, suggests that it is the opposite of nearsightedness, that children with this condition see far-

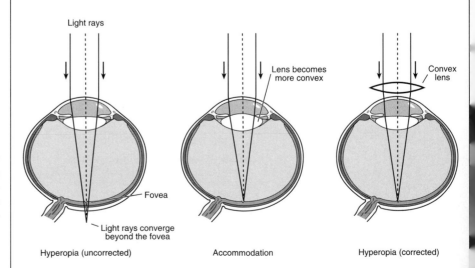

THE OPTICS OF HYPEROPIA. Left: the light rays that come to a focus behind the retina (fovea) may be brought into focus on the retina either by accommodation (center) or by a convex lens (right).

Light rays

Lens becomes more convex

Convex lens

Fovea

Light rays converge beyond the fovea

Hyperopia (uncorrected)

Accommodation

Hyperopia (corrected)

away objects clearly but not things that are near. Unfortunately, it is not that simple. Generally, children with hyperopia see equally well or poorly without glasses (depending on the degree of hyperopia) at all distances.

In discussing myopia, we pretended to look into the eye from the side. When we did, we found that light rays from a distant object came to a focus in front of the retina. If we could also peek into a farsighted eye from the side, we would see that light rays come to a focal point *behind* the retina. In this sense, farsightedness really is the opposite of nearsightedness. It is as if the eye is too short for the way the front part of the eye refracts the light rays.

Accommodation and convergence   To understand hyperopia requires a digression into accommodation and convergence.

The process of focusing for near vision is called *accommodation*. Children's eyes that are normal, or that have been made optically normal with glasses that correct their refractive error, have the remarkable ability to see clearly at all distances.

Optical instruments such as binoculars or cameras cannot change their viewing distance unless the user turns a dial or moves a lever (some cameras automatically focus, but an internal motor "turns the dial"). The eye's focusing "dial" is actually a ring-shaped muscle around the edge of the lens inside the eye. This muscle is part of the *ciliary body*. When the muscle contracts, it makes the ring smaller, which in turn allows the lens to become thicker. A thicker lens has more power—more power to bring close-up objects into focus for clear viewing. When the ciliary muscle relaxes, the lens becomes thinner for clear distant viewing.

ACCOMMODATION. The circular ciliary body contracts and becomes smaller (left). As a result, the lens becomes thicker so that near objects are in focus on the retina (fovea). The opposite is true for distant viewing (right).

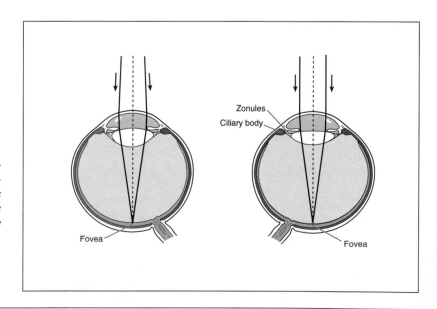

Accommodation does not work alone. When we want to look at something near, the process of accommodation works in conjunction with *convergence*. At the same time that the eyes are bringing an object into focus, they turn in (converge) so that they are both directed at that near object.

This amazing coordination of accommodation and convergence allows us to see near objects not only clearly, but with both eyes at the same time. Our eyes do all of this without any conscious effort on our part.

Hyperopia and strabismus   In children with hyperopia, the light rays from *distant* objects come to a focal point behind the retina, just as the light rays from *near* objects do for those with normal vision. Farsighted people avoid blurred vision at all distances the same way that people with normal vision do when they look at near objects; they accommodate.

> **In order to see clearly at a distance, farsighted children must accommodate and converge the way people with normal eyes do when they are looking at something near.**

With that accommodation there is a fixed degree of convergence, or turning in of the eyes. Without his glasses, Billy must accommodate (unconsciously) to see clearly, and when he is accommodating one of his eyes may turn in. The other eye will be looking straight, at whatever Billy is looking at. This condition, in which the two eyes are looking in different directions, is called *strabismus*. Although not all hyperopic children have strabismus (and not all strabismic children have hyperopia), the crossing of one eye is often the way significant farsightedness makes itself known to parents. This kind of crossing, called *accommodative esotropia*, usually begins around age 2, when children begin to accommodate in order to see fine detail.

> **Without his glasses, Billy must accommodate to see clearly, and when he does, one of his eyes may turn in.**

Other symptoms of hyperopia   Without glasses, hyperopes develop the same symptoms as people with normal vision who read or look at a computer screen for long periods of time. Their eyes become tired or they develop "eyestrain." The reason is that they have to accommodate as much to look at something, say, 14 inches away as those with normal vision do to look at something 6 inches away.

> **Hyperopes wear glasses to see more comfortably, not just better or clearer.**

Hyperopes, including 3-year-old Billy, wear glasses to see more comfortably, not just better or clearer. With hyperopia of mild-to-moderate degree they can see fairly well using accommodation, without glasses, but wearing them makes their eyes feel better.

When hyperopia starts   Hyperopia usually starts in infancy. Indeed, it is normal for babies to be farsighted to some degree. Children need glasses if the farsightedness is very strong, if it is stronger in one eye than the other, or if it causes the eyes to cross in. Otherwise, children who are farsighted do fine without glasses.

Glasses for hyperopia   The lenses that correct this refractive error are thicker in the center, making the eyes appear bigger through the glasses. That is why Billy's eyes always look so big and bright when he wears his glasses. Billy's parents should expect his glasses to get a little stronger until he is 6 or 7, then get a bit weaker until he stops growing. He will probably need glasses (or contact lenses) all his life. But he just might be one of those fortunate few whose hyperopia goes away when they reach their teens.

Presbyopia   Children have a remarkable accommodative ability. They can see things that are only a few inches in front of their noses, clearly and reasonably comfortably, too. From infancy onward, the ability to accommodate gradually decreases, until around age 40 or 45 when we start noticing its loss. This loss of accommodation occurs in all people, whether they have normal, hyperopic, or myopic eyes. The lens becomes less and less flexible, until it can no longer bend to bring near objects into focus.

Billy's father Henry, age 42, has started to have some trouble reading fine print, especially in dim light. His children have been teasing him about getting old, especially since his last birthday. Henry's vision has always been completely normal, but he's beginning to have the same difficulty that nearly everyone develops at about his age: trouble clearly seeing things that are near.

We call Henry's problem *presbyopia* (even though the condition is nearly universal, there is no popular term for it). Presbyopia is not really a refractive error, and it certainly doesn't affect children, but it is so often confused with refractive errors, especially hyperopia, that we will discuss it here.

Presbyopia is related to accommodation: how our eyes change focus to see clearly at near. By age 40 to 45, the nearest point of clear vision is beyond about one foot, even when accommodation is maximal. So Henry is more comfortable holding his newspaper farther away. But as the years go by, it seems as if his arms are getting shorter; he can't seem to move the newspaper far enough away to keep the print in focus. (And even if he could, at that distance the print would be too small to see.) To replace the focusing ability that the lenses in his eyes no longer are capable of, Henry needs a pair of reading glasses. These lenses will be weak magnifying glasses, thicker in the center than at the edge.

At the office, some of Henry's co-workers who wear glasses for distance vision have started wearing bifocals. Bifocals are reading glasses combined with lenses for distance vision; usually the reading segment is in the lower part of the lens. If Henry had bifocals, they would combine the reading glasses on the bottom with clear "window glass" on top. Then he wouldn't have to take off his reading glasses every time he wanted to see something across the room.

As Henry gets older, accommodation will continue to lessen, and his reading glasses will need to be stronger. When he reaches the age

Presbyopia is related to accommodation   how our eyes change focus to see clearly at near.

of 60 or so, all accommodation will be gone, and the prescription won't change anymore.

Henry's presbyopia, of course, is in no way related to Billy's hyperopia. On the other hand, if Billy does not wear his glasses, he may become aware of poor reading vision sooner than his friends of the same age who are not farsighted. Because he has to use some of his accommodation to see even distant objects, he will tend to run out of accommodation as he looks up close.

Astigmatism

Astigmatism has the distinction of being the most confusing refractive error. Astigmatism means the eye focuses light in one meridian more strongly than in the other meridia. Except for blurred vision, there are no signs or symptoms that are characteristic of it. In some cases parents might notice that their child doesn't see as well as they do or as other children do. But astigmatism is usually detected when the child fails a vision screening test. An eye examination is necessary to show that the problem is astigmatism.

If eye doctors were to determine the refractive errors of everyone in the block where Jamie and Billy live, some degree of astigmatism would be found in nearly everyone, even those who see 20/20 without glasses. Most astigmatism is trivial and of no visual significance. Many unnecessary glasses have been prescribed and purchased in the false belief that even a slight astigmatism needs to be corrected, even when the uncorrected vision is normal or nearly so.

Nearly all of Jamie's and Billy's neighbors who are nearsighted or farsighted also have some degree of astigmatism, and the optical correction for it may be incorporated into their glasses. (The glasses that correct astigmatism look the same as those for myopia or hyperopia. Although the front surface of each lens is not symmetrical, that asymmetry is so slight that it cannot be noticed by looking at the glasses.) Astigmatism tends to remain about the same throughout life.

Because astigmatism is so poorly understood, many misconceptions have arisen regarding it. This innocent optical defect has been unjustly blamed for headaches, tired eyes, red eyes, matted eyelashes, poor school performance, and all sorts of other problems.

A little more information about the optics of astigmatism will help you understand this condition.

The optics of astigmatism   In the myopic eye, light from a distant object is focused to a point in front of the retina. In the hyperopic eye, light comes to a focus at a point behind the retina. In the eye with astigmatism, light does not come to a single focal point at all, but, at best, to a focal circle. In fact, the origin of the word astigmatism actually means "no point" *(a = no; stigma = point).*

Like most lenses in optical devices, the lenses in eyeglasses that

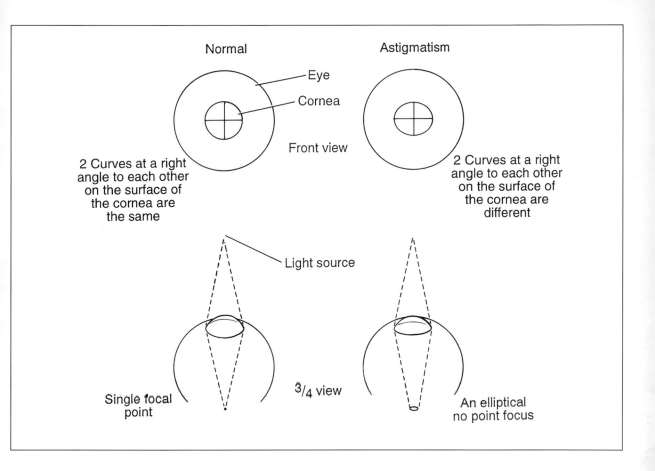

Normal

Eye

Cornea

Front view

2 Curves at a right angle to each other on the surface of the cornea are the same

Astigmatism

2 Curves at a right angle to each other on the surface of the cornea are different

Light source

Single focal point

3/4 view

An elliptical no point focus

THE OPTICS OF ASTIGMATISM. The surface of the cornea is slightly out of round so that light passing through it does not come to a single focal point.

correct myopia and hyperopia have surfaces that are roughly spherical. Imagine a piece of optical glass shaped like a ball. A slice cut from this "ball" would form a lens that would be spherical on one surface and flat on the other. Light going through this lens would come to a focus somewhere, the exact point depending on the diameter of the sphere.

Now imagine a football-shaped piece of optical glass. A slice cut from this glass would form a lens with a certain curve in one direction (say, corresponding to the long axis of the football) and a different curve at an angle 90° from the first curve. Light passing through this lens with its two curves would not come to a single focal point, but at some distance from the lens it would narrow to a circle or ellipse, a no-point focus. This is an astigmatic lens.

In general terms, in an eye with astigmatism, the surface of the cornea is similar to the surface of a slice from a football-shaped piece of glass. The curvature of the surface in one direction is slightly different from the curvature of the surface that is 90° away. That difference in curvature, the "out of round," is usually very small, measured in fractions of a millimeter, but it's enough to make the light reach a no-point focus rather than a focal point. What this translates to for a child with astigmatism is a blur, a reduction of the sharpness of the image that is seen.

A child with astigmatism sees a blur, a reduction of the sharpness of the image.

Astigmatic children live with a blur at all distances, the degree of the blur depending on the severity of the astigmatism.

Differences between astigmatism and other refractive errors
Myopic children experience a blur when looking at something in the distance, and hyperopic children must accommodate more when looking at something up close. Astigmatic children, however, live with the blur at all distances, the degree of blur depending on the severity of the astigmatism.

Let's consider, for example, children whose astigmatism reduces the sharpness of an image from 100% clarity to 90% clarity. The 10% blur would be present at all viewing distances. If they could not read a clock from 20 feet away, they could walk toward it until they could read it.

Though the face and hands would appear larger as they came closer, large enough so they could eventually tell the time, *the 10% blur would still be present.* If these had been myopic children, the details of the clock would not only get larger, they would get clearer too.

This explains to some extent why many children with astigmatism prefer to wear their glasses all the time, while many children with myopia don't. Myopic children whose vision is 20/60 without correction are able to function happily in most situations without glasses. If an object is slightly blurred, they simply move closer to it. Children with astigmatism who can see 20/60 without glasses cannot completely compensate by getting closer.

The genetic link of refractive errors

Should Jamie's mother be surprised that her daughter is becoming nearsighted, or should Billy's parents be surprised that he is farsighted and his cousin Ruth has astigmatism? Not really.

Refractive errors tend to run in families. They are part of a person's genetic makeup. Each child of a parent with a refractive error has about 1 chance in 2 of developing a similar problem. Children with refractive errors will, in turn, tend to pass them on to their own children.

Perhaps someday vision scientists will discover the genes responsible for refractive errors, and eventually they may even be able to correct for them before a child is born. Until that time parents and doctors need to look for the symptoms, and school officials and others need to perform appropriate vision screenings so that optical correction in the form of glasses or contact lenses can be provided when needed.

5

Correcting Vision With Glasses and Contact Lenses

*B*illy's parents *were concerned that the glasses prescribed for their son couldn't possibly be right. After all, he was only two and a half years old when he was first examined. He certainly did not seem to like the eye doctor, especially after he put drops in Billy's eyes. Their son didn't utter a word during the entire exam except a loud "No!" several times, but the doctor seemed confident that Billy was farsighted and that the prescription he was about to give them was correct. How did the doctor know?*

How the doctor determines the right prescription

To find out the kind and amount of refractive error a child has, an eye doctor performs a *refraction*. A refraction is a determination of how a particular eye bends light rays. From the results of the refraction, the doctor can tell what kind of glasses will correct the error in the child's optical system and bring the light rays to a focus on the retina.

Measuring the refraction is not the same as measuring the visual acuity. The visual acuity is the smallest letter or figure that can be seen; the refraction determines the prescription for the spectacles.

The visual acuity is the smallest letter that can be seen (either with or without correction). The refraction determines the eyeglass prescription.

Refractions for older children　When an older child or an adult has a refraction, pairs of lenses are placed before each eye and the patient is asked to look at an an eye chart through them. For each pair of lenses the examiner asks, "Which is better, one or two?" changing them many times until the patient reports that the image is just right.

There are different ways of placing the pairs of lenses in front of the patient's eyes. Some doctors use actual lenses that are kept in a rack. Others prefer a device called a *refractor*, which has the lenses built into it and has dials that are moved to change lenses. Some refractors automatically determine refractive errors. But then those results need to be fine-tuned by asking the age-old question, "Which is better, one or two?"

Refractions for young children   The above techniques cannot work with a preverbal child or one who is too young to cooperate. For these children, a simple instrument called a *retinoscope* allows the refractive error to be determined without any response from the patient. The procedure is called *retinoscopy.*

The retinoscope is a hand-held instrument that projects a streak of light into the pupil. The doctor looks through a hole near the top of the retinoscope, directly along the streak of light, which is reflected off the retina at the back of the eye. To reach the retina the light passes through all of the optical surfaces—the refracting components—of the eye.

If there is a refractive error, the shape or appearance of the reflected light will not be what it should be. The doctor will then hold various lenses of known power in front of the child's eye (while still directing the streak of light into the pupil) until the reflected image is right. The lens that makes the image right identifies the type of refractive error the child has and what strength lenses will correct that refractive error. In principle this technique is very simple, but its proper use is an art that must be perfected through practice.

Retinoscopy is actually based on the movement of the light passed across the pupil, compared to the movement of the reflected image from the retina. If the two move in the same direction, the eye is hyperopic and convex lenses must be added. If they move in opposite directions, the eye is myopic and concave lenses must be added. Astigmatism is determined by comparing the movements in different meridia (i.e., vertically vs. horizontally).

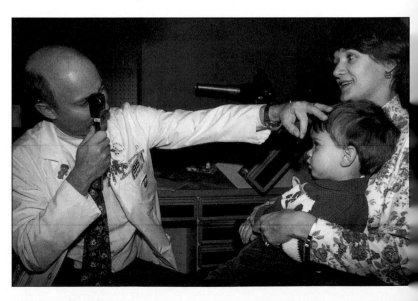

RETINOSCOPY. The doctor is looking through the retinoscope held in the right hand and a lens in his left hand at the reflex from the child's retina. Different lenses are tried until movement of the reflected light is neutralized.

How accurate is retinoscopy?   Billy's father is concerned because he's going to pay a lot of money for Billy's glasses, yet the eye doctor could not ask Billy which lenses were better, the way that his own doctor does with him.

Actually, the use of the retinoscope is very accurate. Without any response from the patient, it can determine a refractive error with such accuracy that the patient can often see nearly 20/20. The glasses may not be perfect, but they should be very close to perfect. In older children and adults, the question "Which is better, one or two?" is asked only to fine-tune the prescription, to give the patient perfect vision. Fortunately for all concerned—children, parents, and eye doctors—when children are old enough to fully appreciate 20/20 vision, they are usually sufficiently cooperative to help in fine-tuning their prescription for glasses.

The use of drops   Billy doesn't like to go to the eye doctor because, as he says, "He's the one with the eyedrops that sting." Perhaps when Billy is older he will be able to have a refraction without them, but for infants and children there is no good alternative for determining the proper glasses.

The drops have two effects that help in the evaluation. The first is obvious: they dilate the pupils. This allows the doctor to perform a thorough examination of the eye's interior with an *ophthalmoscope*. The second effect is important for refraction in infants and children: the drops temporarily paralyze the eye's ability to accommodate. This is called *cycloplegia*. Without it, the constantly changing focus of an eye would make refraction inaccurate.

Sometimes parents ask about side effects from the drops. First of all, the drops blur the vision; in fact, they wouldn't be working if they didn't. Occasionally, crossing of the eyes will become apparent when the pupils dilate. And the child's eyes may be mildly sensitive to light. But all these effects are temporary, usually lasting from 4 to 24 hours. Exactly how long depends on which medication is used, what concentration is chosen, and how many drops are instilled. The effects also depend on the individual child. Blue-eyed children usually stay dilated longer with any given drop than do brown-eyed children.

Rarely, a child may develop flushing, fever, vomiting, behavior changes, or even high blood pressure or abnormal heart rhythm. An allergic response to some eyedrops may cause reddening of the skin around the eyes. It is extremely unusual for any serious side effects to occur or for any treatment to be required other than observation for an hour or so.

Measuring the refractive error   Myopia, hyperopia, and astigmatism—as well as the lenses to correct them—are measured in *diopters*. A diopter is a unit based on the focal length (power) of a lens.

Without glasses, a child with 1 diopter of myopia sees about

Infants and children must have eyedrops for determining the proper glasses. Otherwise, the constantly changing focus of an eye would make refraction inacurate.

20/50. Objects would just begin to blur at 3 or 4 feet away. A child with this low degree of myopia would need 1 diopter of correction in the glasses, which would be worn for board work, perhaps for movies, and, when old enough, for driving.

A 3-diopter myope has about 20/400 vision without correction and would happily wear 3-diopter lenses nearly all the time. If this child removed the glasses, objects would begin to blur at about a foot away and become progressively more blurred as they moved farther away.

The glasses prescription

To explain the glasses prescription a little better, we'll break it down into its components. Each prescription consists of a series of numbers describing the power of the prescribed lenses in diopters.

A 1-diopter lens has a focal length of 1 meter—that is, light from a distant source comes to a focal point 1 meter from the lens; a 2-diopter lens has a focal length of one-half meter, and so on. The larger the number, the stronger the lens and the greater the refractive error that it corrects.

A lens prescription for one eye might be written as follows:

$$-4.25 + 1.50 \times 90$$

−4.25 indicates a minus (concave) lens with a power of 4.25 diopters; it corrects myopia.

+1.50 is the amount of astigmatism, a 1.50 diopter difference in power between the two curves of the cornea.

90 represents 90 degrees, the orientation of one of the curves being measured.

To make matters even more confusing, there are two ways to write this prescription: in "positive" cylinder form:

−4.25 +1.50 x 90

or "negative" cylinder form:

−2.75 −1.50 x 180

To convert negative to positive, add the first two numbers, change the sign of the second, and add (or subtract) 90 from the third.

A progression to larger numbers (stronger glasses) does not mean that the eye is getting worse, but only that the refractive error is getting larger. The most important piece of information regarding the child's eyes is usually not written on the prescription. That is the vision of the child with those glasses.

Visiting the optician   After the prescription has been determined, the preparation of eyeglasses is basically a three-step process: choosing a frame, grinding the lenses, and placing those lenses into the frame.

Opticians are professionals who fill prescriptions. Sometimes eye doctors fill their own prescriptions. Some opticians work in an optical shop; others in the doctor's office. Some opticians have the facilities in their shops to grind the optical glass to the prescribed power; others send the prescription to an optical grinding laboratory to prepare the lenses. Many optical shops keep the most commonly used lenses in house so that the glasses can be prepared fairly quickly.

When Billy's mother was told that he needed glasses, she thought that she would never find a pair of frames to fit his little nose. He was so active that she wondered how glasses would even stay on.

Her concern was reasonable. It is difficult to find frames that properly fit the relatively flat nasal bridge that is so typical of infants and young children. She had to take Billy to several optical shops before she could find a pair of frames that fit him well. But finally the prescription was filled by an optician and put into the frames she selected, and Billy has cheerfully worn them even since.

The single most important factor in determining whether a given frame will fit a young child is the fit at the bridge, the inverted "U" that rests on the sides of the nose. The size of the bridge of the glasses should match the width of the bridge of the nose so that the frames do not slide down. Yet the frame should be far enough forward for the lower portion to not rest on the child's cheek or rub against the lashes. Too often, poorly fitting glasses require the use of elastic straps behind the head. But these may exert constant pressure and create redness and sore spots on the nose.

Flexible hinges on the ear pieces (called "riding bows") can help to hold the glasses up. They also "grow" with the child's face and can help prevent the frames from being broken when they are roughly handled. For very young children, who are often upside down, a useful device is the flexible wrap-around ear piece (called a "comfort cable"). A strap that goes over the top and back of the head may be used for infants.

Parents must expect that glasses will become bent and broken, and that frequent return trips to the optician will be necessary for adjustments and repairs.

The lenses   Nearly all lenses for children these days are made of plastic. Actually, most glasses are not really "glasses"; however, the term is well established and is not likely to change. Plastic lenses scratch a bit more easily than glass lenses, but with reasonable care they should last a year or so. The overwhelming advantage of plastic is that it is about half as heavy as glass. The lighter weight makes it easier for the glasses to stay up on the nose. With children's small noses, plastic lenses are almost a necessity.

Lenses are initially ground in lens blanks, much larger pieces of plastic or glass than what will eventually be fit into the frame. After the frames are selected, these blanks are cut down and edged to fit the size and shape of the frame and to center each lens in front of the appropriate eye. Most optical shops have the facilities to edge prescription lenses and place them in the frames. Before the glasses leave the shop, minor but critical adjustments are made in the nose and ear pieces to allow the glasses to fit comfortably.

How wearing glasses affects a child's life

Should Billy's mother be concerned that his glasses will make him more likely to injure his eyes? After all, he is a typical active 3-year-old boy, carefree and careless. She should not be concerned, and in fact, she should actually be relieved that he is wearing glasses. All prescription lenses, plastic or glass, are required by the United States Food and Drug Administration to be impact-resistant. It is unusual for glasses to injur an eye. Indeed, glasses provide a significant measure of protection from a wide variety of eye injuries that Billy might otherwise sustain in the course of his activities.

Children are children, and wearing glasses will not change their basic nature. Other children can be cruel, however, and glasses can be a focus for teasing. Fortunately, it will become less a problem with time, as more of them develop school-age myopia.

Contact lenses for children

In the last chapter we met Jamie, who was about to get her first glasses for myopia. If Jamie is typical of many young people, she will probably start wanting contact lenses instead of glasses about the time she undergoes that transformation from childhood to young adulthood, when looks become so important to a young person's self-image.

At what age can a child wear contacts? Contact lenses can actually be worn at any age, even in infancy. In fact, they are typically prescribed for babies who have had their natural lenses removed surgically because of cataracts. But most young people who ask for contacts do so for cosmetic reasons: they believe they will look better.

Contact lenses, especially soft contact lenses, require care and maintenance. When children have acquired the motivation, maturity, and discipline necessary for that maintenance regimen, they are old enough for contacts. Typically they are ready when they become teenagers. But if a child is highly motivated for a specific reason—for ballet or soccer, for example—they may be used sooner. It is not necessary to wait until a child's eyes stop growing or changing. The contact lenses will have to be replaced every year or so anyway, even if the eyes do not change.

Types of lenses Contact lenses used to be made of a *hard* plastic material called polymethyl methacrylate (PMMA). Although they had the advantages of correcting astigmatism well and being inexpensive and easy to care for, they had significant disadvantages. They took a long time to get used to, and after years of wear they tended to cause damage to the corneas. These hard lenses are rarely used today.

Most new contact lens wearers are fitted with one of the many varieties of *soft lenses*. These are easier to fit and to wear than hard contacts, and require far less time to get used to. Their disadvantages are that they should be cleaned and sterilized once a day, generally at night. The cost of the supplies for cleaning and sterilization is ongoing, month after month, year after year. The lenses need to be replaced approximately once a year. And most of them do not correct high degrees of astigmatism very well, although special soft lenses that do correct astigmatism (called *toric lenses*) are becoming more successful.

Rigid gas-permeable lenses have some of the advantages of both hard and soft contacts. These lenses are so named because they are made of a rigid plastic that permits oxygen to pass through to reach the cornea. They may be less comfortable than soft lenses, but they require less rigorous maintenance and they share with hard contacts the ability to correct corneal astigmatism. Rigid gas-permeable lenses are becoming more and more popular.

Both soft and gas-permeable lenses are sometimes prescribed for "extended wear," which means that they are not removed at night but are worn continuously for a week or so. We don't generally recommend extended wear except for babies, since the chance of complications is higher than with daily wear lenses.

The possibility of corneal damage   Any contact lens on the surface of the eye is a potential irritant and source of infection. Proper care of the lenses is essential; with appropriate precautions the risk of serious damage to the eye is extremely low.

Contact lenses will not cause injury without some warning sign. The most common indication of trouble is irritation of the eye or redness of the conjunctiva. *Therefore, it is absolutely imperative that the contact lens be removed from any eye that is irritated or red.* If these symptoms do not go away in several hours, the child should be seen promptly by an eye doctor.

If that simple rule is followed, parents and children need not be apprehensive about damage to the eye from contacts. Unfortunately, sometimes the pressure to continue wearing them for the big game or the big social event causes symptoms to be ignored, with potentially disastrous consequences.

Correcting refractive errors without glasses

Most people who wear glasses or contact lenses do so for myopia (nearsightedness). Wouldn't it be nice if there were some way to prevent the progression of myopia once it starts, or even to reverse it? Jamie's parents would do anything to free their daughter from the need to wear glasses the rest of her life.

One of the neighbors told them that simply wearing contact lenses will retard or stop the progression of myopia. Unfortunately, there is no evidence to substantiate that belief. The fact that most contact lenses for myopia are initially fitted during the middle teenage years, when the progression of myopia typically slows or stops anyway, explains how this erroneous idea could have begun.

Reversing myopia with contact lenses   Some optometrists say they can prevent the progression of myopia or even reverse it with a process called *orthokeratology*. This process involves deliberately misfitting a contact lens to change the shape of the cornea and, thereby, the eye's refractive power. It is similar in concept to reducing the size of the foot by fitting the shoe too tightly. The cornea, however, retains its new shape for only a few days, returning to its original shape soon after the misfit lens has been removed.

Correcting refractive errors with surgery   In recent years, some ophthalmologists have advocated surgical treatment to correct refractive errors.

In the 1970s a procedure called *radial keratotomy* (RK) was developed to reduce or eliminate myopia. Usually four to eight incisions are made from near the center of the cornea outward to its edge. As these incisions heal, the cornea flattens, changing its refraction to lessen the degree of myopia. The procedure has been performed on several hundred thousand patients in this country. Most have been pleased with the outcome, but some have not. Though rare, there have been significant complications that have resulted in loss of vision.

Within the past several years a new type of laser, called the excimer laser, has been used to alter the shape of the cornea. Its major advantage is improved predictability of refractive change. Excimer corneal surgery (called *photorefractive keratectomy*, or PRK) has largely supplanted RK as the technique of choice for surgically correcting refractive errors.

There are also other, less common, surgical procedures for treating refractive errors. All are still investigational, as of this writing. We endorse refractive surgery only in special circumstances and believe that anyone considering it would be wise to learn about all the risks. For children, especially, we do not advocate this type of surgery.

MUSCLE PROBLEMS

Parents instinctively seek eye contact with their infants from the time they're born, and infants respond as if to a physical need. Eye contact, psychologists tell us, plays a central role in the process of bonding. When Susie can't reliably look into her parents' eyes, they can be quite disconcerted. They may think she is blind, when in fact she is just cross-eyed, and they were seeking contact with the wrong eye.

Nearly all of us know someone who has an eye or eyes that cross in or turn out. Perhaps we ourselves were told by our mothers that we were cross-eyed when we were babies and grew out of it.

The subject of "crossed eyes" and related disorders is complicated. In this section, we will explain how these disorders are classified, how they affect a child's vision, and how they can be treated.

Strabismus Terminology and Classification

o Named by the direction of the deviating eye

> The terms ending in –tropia indicate an actual deviation:
>
> **ESOTROPIA** *the eye turns in (crosses); also called* CONVERGENT STRABISMUS
> **EXOTROPIA** *the eye turns out (wall eye); also called* DIVERGENT STRABISMUS
> **HYPERTROPIA** *the eye turns up*
> **HYPOTROPIA** *the eye turns down*

> The terms ending in –phoria indicate a *tendency* for an eye to deviate, which is controlled by fusion:
>
> **ESOPHORIA** *the eye tends to turn inward*
> **EXOPHORIA** *the eye tends to turn outward*
> **HYPERPHORIA** *the eye tends to turn upward*
> **HYPOPHORIA** *the eye tends to turn downward*

o Named by how frequently the eye deviates

> **INTERMITTENT** *sometimes both eyes are straight; sometimes one deviates*
> **CONSTANT** *the eye always deviates*

o Named by which eye deviates

> **RIGHT** *the right eye always deviates*
> **LEFT** *the left eye always deviates*
> **ALTERNATING** *sometimes the right eye deviates and sometimes the left eye deviates*

o Named by the age of onset

> **CONGENITAL** *present at birth or soon after (difficult to distinguish from* INFANTILE*)*
> **INFANTILE** *onset before 1 year of age*
> **CHILDHOOD** *onset after 1 or 2 years of age*

o Named by the known or presumed cause

> **ACCOMMODATIVE** *related to accommodation, the process of focusing at different distances*
> **SENSORY** *resulting from poor vision in one or both eyes*
> **IDIOPATHIC** *resulting from an unknown cause*
> **SECONDARY** *related to a neurologic or orbital disorder*

o Named by the pattern of deviation

> **COMITANT** *the angle of deviation is the same in all positions of gaze*
> **INCOMITANT** *the angle of deviation is different in some positions*
> **A PATTERN** *the eyes are more convergent in upgaze and more divergent in downgaze, like the letter A*
> **V PATTERN** *the eyes are more convergent in downgaze and more divergent in upgaze, like the letter V*

6

An Introduction to Strabismus

In the Introduction we met Heather, the adorable two-year-old whose right eye suddenly began to turn in. Her parents wanted to know why the eye doctor prescribed glasses and why he made her wear a patch on her good eye. Then he recommended surgery, and they did not understand how that would help her eyesight.

To understand Heather's problems and their treatment, we must look at the way normal eyes work together. Then we will discuss each of the individual disorders and how they are handled.

How normal eyes work together

Most infants do not have perfectly straight eyes at birth. Research has shown that, in fact, their eyes often turn out. But by the time they are 2 or 3 months old the eyes are a perfect team, moving together, looking left or right and up or down in unison regardless of how far or in which direction they are focused. Such is the case, at least in the vast majority of newborns.

This alignment is achieved more or less naturally as long as each individual eye is otherwise normal and has good vision. The precision of eye coordination is amazing, within a fraction of a degree for each eye. It is what allows for the development of *binocular vision*, or binocularity, the formation of a single image from visual information from both eyes. All of this is accomplished with the aid of our biological computer—the brain—and its connections.

As a result of binocular vision, the vast majority of us acquire a fringe benefit: stereoscopic vision, or *stereopsis*. Steropsis is a unique and highly specialized type of depth perception that helps us to judge how far or how close something is. We have it because our two eyes are separated from each other by about 2 inches, so each provides a slightly different perspective. The brain takes the visual information from each eye and instantly computes the distance of the object we are looking at.

Stereoscopic vision is most useful when there is no other visual information from which depth can be judged—for instance, if one wanted to know the distance of a white object in a totally white room that is uniformly lit so that there are no shadows. It also allows us to perceive the depth illusion in 3-D movies and in some eye tests. In most real-life circumstances, people who have grown up without stereopsis function quite normally using monocular clues for depth perception. Such people even fly private airplanes and play professional sports.

Most people who have grown up without stereoscopsis function quite normally using monocular clues for depth perception.

A child's innate desire to use both eyes together is fairly strong. The ability to bring the eyes into alignment and to use them together for single binocular vision is called *fusion*.

What is strabismus?

If the eyes are not properly aligned, each eye looks in a different direction. Strabismus is a general term for any misalignment of the eyes, irrespective of the direction or the degree of misalignment. One of the eyes is presumably looking directly at the object of interest and sees that object clearly. The other eye, the deviating eye, is not looking directly at the object.

Double vision   If strabismus develops in an adult, the result may be double vision: two images of the same object. One image is clear; the second image, though less clear, can be very annoying. The clear image is produced from the information received by the eye that is looking directly at the object. The unclear image is produced from information received by the deviating eye. You can intentionally cause double vision by pushing gently on one of your eyes through the lid. Immediately a second, blurry image will appear next to the "real" one.

Suppression   Strabismus usually starts in early childhood, typically before age 4 or so. Young children have a remarkable ability to "turn off" or suppress the image from the deviating eye, preventing double vision. Therefore, most young children who develop strabismus do not have double vision, and their ability to suppress the second image remains throughout life. But older children or adults who develop strabismus may not be able to suppress the image from the deviating eye. Sometimes they are troubled by double vision for the rest of their lives.

Does one eye deviate, or do both?   Children with strabismus use only one eye at a time. If the child is looking with the right eye, an observer might say that the left eye is deviating (not looking at the object). Then if the child decides (consciously or subconsciously) to look with the left eye, the observer might say that the right eye is deviating. In each case the observer thinks that the deviating eye is the defective one, that it is the eye needing treatment. But actually neither eye alone is at fault; the eyes are misaligned *in relation to each other.*

The relationship between strabismus and vision

What is the relationship between poor vision and strabismus, and which comes first? Actually, either may cause or contribute to the other.

Strabismus as the cause of poor vision   As we said before, a child up to about age 7 can suppress the image from the deviating eye to avoid seeing double. But this suppression is a mixed blessing. Over time, the eye that is suppressed may lose vision, may "forget" how to see due to lack of use. Before the strabismus started, the child may have had equally good vision in both eyes. In a relatively short time, usually weeks or months, one eye may be seeing worse than the other.

This loss of vision in an otherwise healthy eye is known as *amblyopia,* and it is sometimes called "lazy eye." In this example the strabismus caused the amblyopia. The typical treatment for amblyopia is to force the deviating eye to be used—retrain it to see—by *patching* (covering) the preferred eye until the vision of the two eyes is equal. Even then, the strabismus will probably persist. If so, it may require treatment—sometimes glasses, but often surgery.

Poor vision as the cause of strabismus   Sometimes poor vision in one eye can lead to strabismus. A deviation of this type is sometimes called a *sensory strabismus.*

A pair of normal eyes works together like a well-trained team of horses. But if one eye doesn't see well, it might gradually deviate because it does not have enough visual information to keep it aligned with its teammate. In infants, the deviating eye tends to turn in (sensory esotropia). In older children and adults, it tends to drift out (sensory exotropia). At all ages, the deviating eye may be higher than the other eye.

If we could somehow restore that eye's vision quickly, before it drifted too far, the improved vision might allow it to get back in line again, to work with the other eye in a normal fashion. On the other hand, if the eye has drifted too far or if it has been too long since it worked with the other eye, restoring its vision might not cause it to straighten. The deviating eye would have to be moved back into alignment by some other means, perhaps surgery. Although surgery can control sensory deviations, they may recur after a time. Sometimes glasses can help, especially if a child with sensory esotropia is farsighted in the good eye. Unfortunately, aligning a deviating eye with surgery does not restore its vision.

Visual function in children with strabismus

How well do children with strabismus function? Does it affect their schoolwork or their ability to play baseball or ride their bicycles? Does it put a "strain" on one eye and cause tired eyes in activities such as reading?

The effect of strabismus on binocularity   Normal binocular vision develops naturally during infancy. Children learn to use both eyes together simultaneously, integrating visual information from each eye to produce a single mental picture in the brain.

If a constant strabismus starts at birth or in the first several months of life, it is impossible to use both eyes together. The infant may learn to see well with each eye alone, alternating fixation. But for binocular vision to develop the eyes must be aligned, usually by surgery, before 1 or 2 years of age. And even then, binocular vision is not achieved to the same high degree that it is in children without strabismus.

Most strabismus develops between birth and age 4. By the first birthday, children have learned to use both eyes together, so if strabismus starts then they are initially, but briefly, aware of seeing double. If such children cannot blink or look somewhere else and regain the proper alignment, they may begin to suppress the vision from the deviating eye.

Once suppression has eliminated the double vision, children function quite happily. They may use their preferred eye or alternate from one eye to the other, but in either case they are seeing well. Double vision is eliminated by suppression. It is true that they have lost their stereoscopic vision, but most children learn to judge depth with one eye using monocular clues and are able to function as well as any other child. When they are older they should be able to play baseball just like the other children.

The effect of strabismus on peripheral vision   Will the child's peripheral vision be normal? In other words, will the child who has suppressed vision from one eye be able to see cars or tacklers or tigers coming from that side? Surprisingly, the child's peripheral vision is nearly normal. The car, the tackler, or the tiger will be seen almost as well as by any other child. The reason is that only the central vision, the part of the visual field that is directed straight ahead, is suppressed in the deviating eye. Children whose eyes turn outward may actually have wider-than-normal visual fields.

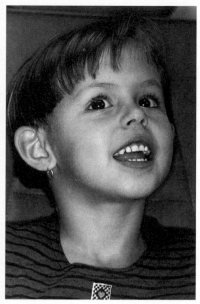

ABNORMAL HEAD POSITION TO COMPENSATE FOR STRABISMUS. A child may prefer a left face turn because the eyes are not straight unless they are turned to the right. Abnormal head postures can include head tilting to either side and chin elevation or depression, as well. They are particularly apparent when the child views interesting objects that are hard to see.

Head positions that compensate for strabismus

There are some uncommon kinds of strabismus in which one or both eyes do not move the normal full range in one or several directions so that the eyes are not aligned in straight-ahead gaze. Infants and children with these types of strabismus may hold their head in an abnormal position, turning their face to the left or the right, tilting their head to one side or the other, or raising or lowering their chin so that both eyes can work together.

Children who are unable to raise one eye to the straight-ahead position, for example, would almost certainly raise their chin to look straight ahead, because downgaze is the only position where both eyes are aligned. This abnormal head posture, driven by the natural striving for binocular vision, is often the sign that is noticed by the family. When the child uses a head position that allows the eyes to be aligned, both eyes usually develop good vision and binocular function is often normal.

When children with an abnormal head posture look away from the preferred position, they are not as happy. In general, it's best to allow them to hold their head as they choose. But physicians and parents should realize that an abnormal head position may be a sign of an eye problem.

How the different kinds of strabismus are classified

Sometimes parents are confused because different doctors chose different words to describe the same thing. Similar confusion might come from describing the same car as a red car, a hatchback, a two-door, or a stick-shift; all might be correct. So it is with strabismus, which can be classified in a variety of ways.

By the direction of the deviating eye   This is the most common (and useful) way to classify strabismus. The deviating eye may be turned in toward the nose, or *convergent*; that condition is called *esotropia*, and the child who has it is said to be cross-eyed. The deviating eye may be turned out toward the ear, or *divergent*; that is called *exotropia*, and the child who has it is sometimes said to be wall-eyed. Finally, the deviating eye may be higher than the other, called *hypertropia*, or lower, called *hypotropia*.

These terms, all ending in –tropia, refer to an actual or manifest strabismus. Some children merely have a tendency for the eyes to turn, and the terms for those conditions begin the same but end in –phoria (*esophoria*). Phorias are not easily seen because they are controlled by fusion.

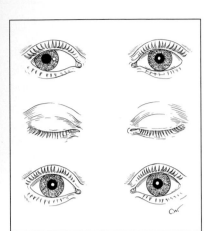

INTERMITTENT STRABISMUS is sometimes controlled as a phoria and sometimes manifest as a tropia. In this example, an intermittent right exotropia comes under control after a blink.

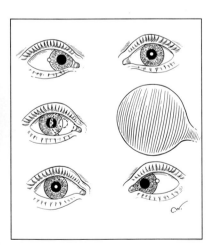

ALTERNATING STRABISMUS. Top: the right eye is esotropic. Center: covering the fixing left eye may force the right eye to move out and assume fixation. Bottom: the cover removed; if the right eye can then maintain fixation with the left eye turned in, the child has an alternating strabismus.

By how often the eye deviates Any deviation may be *intermittent* or *constant*, and those words are sometimes used with the name for the type of strabismus: for example, *intermittent exotropia* or *constant hypertropia*. Because intermittent deviations, by definition, are sometimes manifest (tropias) and sometimes controlled by fusion (phorias), they are occasionally called "phoria-tropias." Intermittent deviations occur more often, or more obviously, when the child is tired or ill.

By which eye deviates If one eye always deviates and the other is always used for looking, the strabismus is sometimes classified with reference to the deviating eye. If only the right eye turns in, and never the left, this would be called a *right esotropia*.

If the child looks sometimes with one eye, sometimes with the other, alternating fixation, the strabismus may be labeled to reflect this: for example, *alternating esotropia*.

By the age of onset If the strabismus starts at birth or soon after, it is called *congenital*. If it starts within the first several months of life, before the child reaches 1 year of age, it is referred to as *infantile*. Congenital and infantile esotropia are often considered together because it is often hard to know exactly when the deviation began. Exotropia usually begins after age 1 or 2 and is sometimes called *childhood exotropia*.

By the known or presumed cause In most cases, strabismus has no apparent underlying cause and is therefore called *idiopathic*. Some children develop esotropia because of convergence from overactive accommodation; this is an *accommodative esotropia*. Deviations resulting from poor vision are called *sensory strabismus*. *Secondary* deviations are those with a known cause, for example, a neurologic or orbital disorder. *Consecutive* deviations are those that follow surgery for an opposite deviation—for example, a consecutive exotropia following esotropia surgery.

By the amount of deviation in various gazes No matter what type of strabismus the child has, the eyes will usually deviate about the same amount no matter what the direction of gaze; *that is, there is a constant angle of deviation regardless of the direction in which the child is looking.* That constancy of the angle of deviation is called *comitance*. Most strabismus in childhood is *comitant*. But sometimes the angle of the deviation changes with different directions of gaze. In such cases the strabismus is called *incomitant*.

Treatment strategies for strabismus

Before any kind of treatment is begun, if one eye has better vision than the other, the usual first step is to try to make both eyes see equally well, so that either one can be used for looking. This usually involves patching the better eye and often using glasses too.

Some parents may find the outcome of equalizing the vision disconcerting. Initially only one eye deviated, but once the vision is equal in both eyes, the better eye may also deviate. The child alternates—that is, looks alternately with one eye, then the other. After all, if the two eyes see equally well, there is no reason to prefer either one.

In some cases, glasses may align the eyes. Children with small angle asymptomatic deviations may simply be observed. Eye muscle surgery is considered in cases with larger deviations, symptoms of double vision, abnormal head positions, or threatened loss of fusion.

7   Testing for Alignment

I n this chapter we will describe some of the most useful examination techniques for diagnosing alignment problems. Most of them apply to all types of strabismus.

Testing positions

In daily living, a person's face is usually directed toward whatever he or she is looking at. The straight-ahead position is therefore the most important, both for distance and for near viewing. This is called the *primary position.*

Alignment is usually assessed in more than one position of gaze, depending on how cooperative the child is. The primary position is tested first, then the *secondary positions,* which are roughly 30° to the left, right, up and down from the primary position. (For testing, the face is moved while the child is still looking at a toy or the television screen.) In certain circumstances, eye alignment is checked in the *oblique* positions as well; for these measurements, the child's face is turned up-and-left or down-and-right, or even tilted toward either shoulder. Depending on the type of misalignment, all these positions may be important in planning treatment.

The cover test

The most useful test of alignment, and one of the most accurate, is the *cover test.* With the child's attention securely fixed on an object such as a toy or a TV screen, the examiner uses a hand or a black paddle to cover and uncover each eye in turn, watching for movement of the eye that is not covered.

First the cover is placed over the right eye and then removed. If there is no strabismus, both eyes will continue to be directed toward the object when the cover is removed (think of an imaginary line connecting the object to the fovea of each eye). The left eye will not move because both eyes are already be directed at the object. But what if the left eye is turned in or out? Then, covering the right eye will usually result in the left eye moving to look straight at the object. Because either eye may be turned, the cover test must be repeated for both eyes.

The cover test can be done with near or distant objects. It is particularly useful when the eyes are only slightly turned in or out, since the movement of the turned eye (to look at the object when the other eye is covered) will be easier to see than the misalignment itself.

At any age, a person with misaligned eyes will use the stronger eye, allowing the weaker eye to drift. That is usually the case even when the vision of the two eyes is only slightly different. Children who see equally well with both eyes often alternate the use of their eyes.

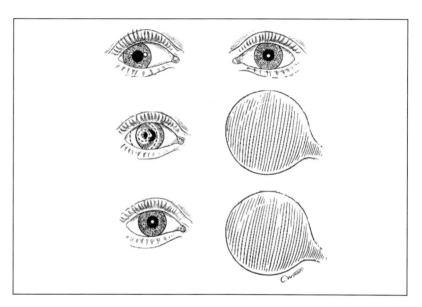

THE COVER TEST. Top: Because children who have strabismus almost always use their better eye, even small angle strabismus in one eye often indicates poor vision in the eye that turns. Center: The right eye centers when the left eye is covered. Bottom: We suspect that the right eye does not see as well as the left eye, especially if the right eye drifts again when the cover is removed.

Two modifications of the cover test

The cross cover test   The cover test can detect an actual deviation: a *tropia*. But when a deviation is latent—called a *phoria*—the eyes tend to drift but are held in alignment by fusion. Latent deviations may be difficult to see even with the cover test. (They may be noticed by looking behind the cover or by watching for movement of the eye as it is uncovered.) A way to make them easier to see is to move the cover from one eye directly to the other, so that the two eyes are never allowed to look together. This modification is called the *cross cover* (or *alternate cover*) test.

The prism cover test   Because they bend light, prisms can be

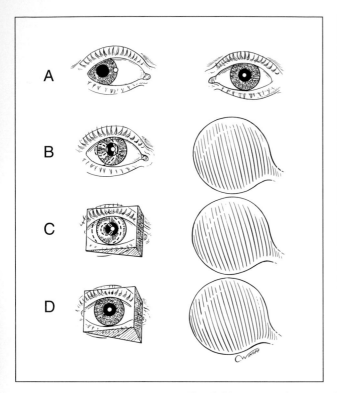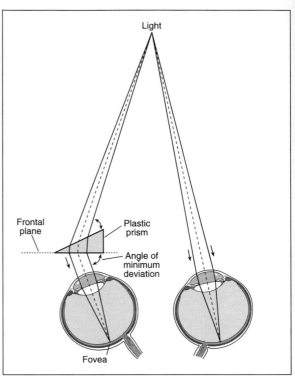

THE PRISM COVER TEST . Left: A. The child is seen to have a right exotropia. B: The cover test shows movement of the right eye to fixate when the left eye is covered. C: A small prism introduced before the right eye begins to neutralize the deviation. D: The correct prism has been introduced, and no more movement is seen when the cover is alternated between eyes. Right. The diagram shows how the prism eliminates movement on cover testing by aligning rays of light from the fixation target with the fovea in the exotropic right eye. The size of the prism gives a measurement of the exotropia.

used to measure the angle of the strabismus. For this test, different strength prisms are held before the eye(s) until one is found that perfectly matches the deviation. After the image through the prism is aligned with the fovea of the deviating eye, there will be no movement on cross cover testing.

Testing the corneal light reflex

Some children, especially those who are very young, will not pay enough attention to the toys used in testing to allow for reliable cover testing. Their eye alignment can be assessed using the corneal light reflex.

The examiner simply shines a penlight at the child's nasal bridge. If the eyes are straight, the reflection of the light will fall near the center of each pupil. But if the left eye is turned, the light will fall to one side of the left pupil—to the outside if the eye is crossed in, and to the inside if the eye is turned out. How far the light is dis

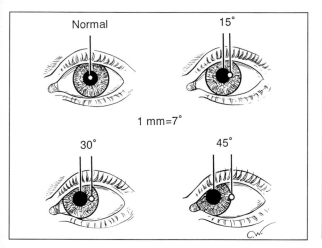

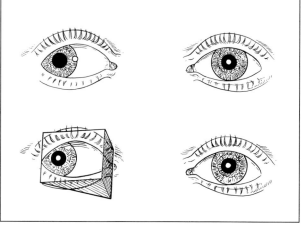

THE HIRSHBERG TEST. The extent to which the corneal light reflex is displaced from the center of the pupil provides an approximation of the angular size of the deviation (in this example a left esotropia).

THE KRIMSKY TEST. The right exotropia in the top picture is measured by the size of the prism required to center the pupillary reflexes (bottom picture).

placed is a rough measure of how far the eye is turned. This test is sometimes called the *Hirshberg test.*

Just as prisms can be combined with the cover test, they can also be combined with the light reflex test. When prisms are used to center the light reflex in each pupil, the test is called the *Krimsky test.*

❧

The accuracy of measurements is generally greatest with the prism cover test, intermediate with the Krimsky test, and least with the Hirshberg test.

Examining eye movements

Eye alignment and movement are closely related. So, in addition to testing alignment, it is important to assess how well the eyes move in various directions. A left eye that can't move to the left will tend to be crossed, maybe in all positions, but especially when the child looks to the left with the right eye. (Children may compensate by turning their face to the left so that their eyes are both to the right, because in that position they can use both eyes together.)

As the eyes are rotated into the different positions, any asymmetry of movement is watched for. In this way the functioning of all six muscles in each eye can be assessed. Sometimes it's hard to coax young children to move their eyes into all the positions for testing. A combination of toys, games, and bribes may be necessary.

Testing for suppression: the Worth 4-dot test

Many children with a misaligned eye tend to suppress vision in that eye in order to avoid seeing double. This tendency can be identified with the Worth 4-dot test, which uses four lights—two green, one red, and one white—and a pair of red-green glasses. Children as young as 2 are sometimes able to point to the lights even if they can't count or name colors.

The test is given with both the child's eyes open. A child looking with only the right eye through the red lens will see the red light and the white light, but not the two green ones. Similarly, a child who is looking with only the left eye through the green lens will see the two green lights and the white light, but not the red one.

The test is simple but clever. A child who is suppressing the left eye will say there are two lights, and one who is suppressing the right eye will say there are three lights. Only the child who's using both eyes will see all four.

Like other tests of vision, this one is easier for young children to do at close range, but it is more sensitive if it's done at a distance.

Stereoscopic vision

Children with misaligned eyes tend to have poor stereopsis. This can be determined with various tests, most using polarized sunglasses to look at stereoscopic pictures or circles. The images appear elevated to people with normal stereoscopic vision. Because stereoscopic vision is frequently abnormal in children who have other vision problems, these tests are sometimes used in vision screening. Poor stereopsis alone rarely causes any functional problem for a child who is used to it.

Now that we have reviewed the classification and examination of strabismus in general, we can proceed to a discussion of the specific deviations. These are the subjects of the next three chapters.

8

Esotropia:
Eyes That Turn In

Esotropia, commonly called "crossed eyes," is the most frequently encountered form of strabismus. There are three broad categories of esotropia: congenital (also called infantile), accommodative, and sensory. Sensory esotropia was discussed briefly in Chapter 6 ("Poor vision as a cause of strabismus"). The other two, which are far more common, will be the focus of this chapter.

Congenital esotropia

In spite of its name, congenital esotropia rarely starts at birth; it is generally first noted at several months of age. Thus it is sometimes called *infantile esotropia*, which is actually a more accurate term. This form occurs frequently in children who have cerebral palsy, hydrocephalus, or developmental delay, and is less common (about 1 in 100) among otherwise normal infants. Usually there is no family history, but it is more likely if other family members have the same condition. Infantile esotropia is idiopathic.

In nearly all cases, the angle of crossing is fairly large so that the deviation is easily seen, at least by 6 months of age when the infant is sitting well and looking at the world. About half of these infants

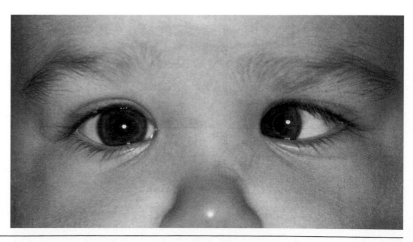

CONGENITAL ESOTROPIA. Typically beginning during the first 6 months of life, this large deviation is probably better termed infantile esotropia. Note the displacement of the corneal light reflex in the left eye, indicating approximately a 20 degree esotropia by the Hirshberg method.

fixate alternately with each eye, so both eyes learn to see well. In the other half, one eye is preferred for looking and the eye that is not used becomes amblyopic ("lazy").

Treatment: Treatment begins with covering the good eye with a patch in order to force the use of the weak eye and strengthen its vision. After vision in the two eyes has been equalized, the esotropia nearly always remains, and surgery is needed to correct it.

It is generally felt that it is better to move each eye half the distance needed to correct the deviation than to operate on just one eye. Most ophthalmologists, at least in North America, prefer to do the surgery when the child is between the ages of 6 and 18 months, when there may still be time for the development of some binocularity. In most cases the eyes straighten immediately after surgery and the child begins to use both eyes together. Many parents report a jump in performance soon afterward, with the child acquiring some new skill or reaching some new milestone in development.

Nearly always, the esotropia remains after the vision is equalized by patching, and surgery is needed to correct it.

About half of these children will have eyes that remain essentially straight indefinitely. They learn to use their eyes together, though not quite as well as those who have never had strabismus. They do not acquire the high degree of stereopsis needed to pass the test to become fighter pilots, for example, but in other respects their eyes are normal for the rest of their lives.

In the other half of these children, the eyes do not remain aligned. Strabismus of some sort appears again, usually showing up months to years later. The esotropia may recur (often as accommodative esotropia, which can be controlled with glasses; if not, more surgery may be required). Less often, exotropia develops and may also require more surgery, perhaps years later.

Sometimes, either before or after surgery, one or both eyes begin to turn upward. This *hypertropia* is most likely to start when the child is between 1 and 4 years of age. There are several types, which will be discussed in Chapter 10.

Pseudoesotropia in infants. Parents and grandparents may initially expect the crossing to disappear on its own. This is a misconception that arises because many infants appear to have crossed eyes when in fact they do not; this *pseudoesotropia* does disappear as the infant gets older. True esotropia, unfortunately, does not disappear.

Nearly all infants appear to have crossed eyes *(see photo at right).* Older children and adults have an equal amount of white space (the sclera) on each side of the colored iris. But in infants, the sclera is partly hidden by their flat, wide nasal bridges. Eventually, the head gets larger, the eyes move farther apart and the bridge of the nose becomes more prominent, in effect pulling together the skin between the eyes and exposing more of the sclera.

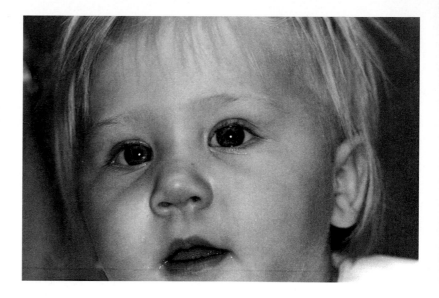

PSEUDOESOTROPIA. Because this photograph shows the child looking slightly to his left, the right eye looks turned in. However, the corneal light reflex from the flash camera is centered in each pupil, indicating normal alignment.

Accommodative esotropia

The most common esotropia is the type called "accommodative," which is intimately related to hyperopia (farsightedness). Accommodative esotropia typically starts at about the age of 2, but the child may be as young as 6 months or as old as 5 years. The deviation may be intermittent at first, but it usually becomes constant soon afterward. Many children begin to prefer one eye, so amblyopia is likely to develop in the deviating eye. If the esotropia begins during an illness or after a fall, the parents may think it was caused by the illness or injury; however, the two occurrences are really just a coincidence.

Up to about age 40, the normal eye has the remarkable ability of *accommodation,* which provides focusing power to bring the focal point forward toward the retina to obtain clearer vision. When people with normal eyes look at something near, each eye accommodates to see the near object. Farsighted (hyperopic) people must use exactly the same process to clear their vision for distant objects—and even more for near ones.

If the amount of hyperopia is large enough, the amount of accommodation needed to see clearly will cause so much convergence that one eye will turn in.

Whenever the eyes accommodate, whether to look at something near or to clear the distance vision in hyperopia, the eyes have a tendency to converge, or turn in. If the degree of the hyperopia is large enough, the amount of accommodation needed to see clearly—even at a distance—will cause so much convergence that one eye will turn in.

Moderately farsighted children, in order to see clearly at a distance, must accommodate and converge as much as people with normal eyes do when they are looking at something near. In doing so, they become esotropic. If they wear glasses to correct the farsightedness, the lenses do the focusing and there is no need for the eyes

ACCOMMODATIVE ESOTROPIA. Top: the right eye of this farsighted child turns in when he looks with the left eye without glasses. Bottom: with glasses on, the child's eyes are straight. The pupils have been dilated for examination. (Photos courtesy Ken Wright, M.D.)

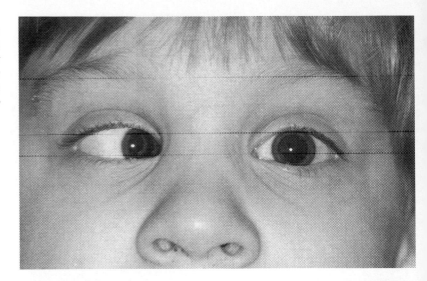

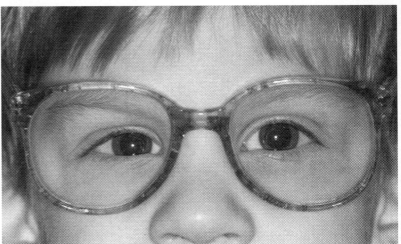

to accommodate or to converge. Happily, the eyes are straight, but only as long as the glasses are worn. (Some farsighted children are fortunate to have an unusual capacity to control their alignment when accommodating, and as a result manage to avoid esotropia.)

Most children are at least slightly farsighted for their first 6 years or so. But in about 98% of them the hyperopia is so mild that the little accommodation needed to see clearly does not cause excessive convergence. The eyes remain straight, with no esotropia. In the other 2% the hyperopia is strong enough to cause too much convergence when the child accommodates to see clearly, and esotropia results. Accommodative esotropia often runs in families. But it isn't inherited; it's the hyperopia that is inherited.

Treatment: The first step is to determine the degree of hyperopia (along with any astigmatism) that is present and to prescribe corrective glasses. If the child has amblyopia, treatment for that condition may be started at this time, or it may be started at a later visit.

As soon as the child begins to wear the glasses, the esotropia decreases, with the full effect taking place within about a month. For most children with accommodative esotropia, glasses eliminate the esotropia completely, or nearly so, and no surgery is needed. If a noticeable esotropia remains even when the child is wearing the proper glasses, the ophthalmologist and the parents may decide to correct the remaining esotropia with eye muscle surgery.

For most children with accommodative esotropia, glasses eliminate the esotropia completely, or nearly so, and no surgery is needed.

The child will need to wear glasses as long as the hyperopia is great enough to cause esotropia when they aren't worn. Most children with accommodative esotropia will probably wear glasses or contact lenses as long as they live. They do so willingly; they see more comfortably when the glasses relieve the need to accommodate and they may appreciate the restoration of binocularity.

They will probably wear glasses or contact lenses as long as they live.

The hyperopia will likely increase until about the first grade, then decrease a bit over the next decade. In a few children the hyperopia just gradually goes away; by the time they are teenagers these lucky few no longer need glasses.

Esotropia at near   Because it's normal to accommodate when looking at something up close, it's not surprising that accommodative esotropia is sometimes worse at near. In fact, about half of all children with accommodative esotropia have an increased angle of crossing when they read.

A few children may actually have eyes that are straight when they are looking at a distance and cross only when they are looking at something close. In these cases, the problem may be difficult to see, since the crossing may be hidden by what the child is looking at—a book, for example. The deviation is typically noticed at mealtime. When the child's head is up and the eyes are fully visible, the family can see the eye turning inward.

Treatment: If the added crossing for near vision is mild, it may require no added treatment. Children who are mildly farsighted and whose eyes are straight for distance vision and cross only slightly at near may simply be observed. Children who are very farsighted may get enough relief from their regular glasses even when looking up close.

Bifocal lenses are the classic treatment for the added crossing at near. Just like the bifocals prescribed for presbyopia, these have added focusing power in the lower segments of the lenses. The upper segments contain the regular distance prescription.

It's surprising how easily children adapt to bifocals; indeed, they seem to take to them much better than adults do! Of course, if they happen to look at something up close through the upper segments of the lenses, the crossing may momentarily reappear. And they occasionally complain of double vision from the line between the lens segments (which should ideally be positioned even with their pupils). But such problems are remarkably minor. As the children get older, the added crossing at near may gradually decrease and the strength of the bifocals can be decreased as well. In some cases, they can eventually be discontinued altogether.

Partially accommodative esotropia   Some children with accommodative esotropia achieve only partial control of their crossing when they wear their farsighted correction (even with bifocals). The esotropia is much less when the glasses are worn, but some crossing remains.

The problem can occur in several different ways.

o A 2-year-old begins to cross an eye, is found to be farsighted, and is given the correct glasses. But even with glasses the child's eyes still cross badly enough that surgery is required. This was the case with little Heather, whose story we have been following (Introduction, Chapter 6). Some specialists believe this sequence is more likely if treatment is delayed beyond a few weeks or months after the crossing begins.

o An esotropia that initially responds to glasses can later "deteriorate" so that glasses no longer completely straighten the eyes. It isn't known why this change occurs, but fortunately it doesn't happen very often. Surgery is usually successful.

o A child requires surgery for esotropia either because glasses aren't needed or because they simply don't make the eyes straight. After the eyes have been successfully aligned by surgery, the esotropia may recur, usually to a much smaller degree. This time the glasses can control the esotropia. Actually, this type of partially accommodative esotropia occurs fairly often.

More about treatment

It's easy to see that esotropia and its treatment can be confusing, especially when children have a combination of several different types. Some children may begin with glasses, progress to bifocals, then eventually need surgery anyway. One question some parents ask is, "If surgery is needed to correct the crossing that remains since my child has started to wear glasses, why not move the muscles a bit more and eliminate all of the crossing with surgery? Wouldn't my child then have straight eyes without glasses?"

That is a logical question. In a few cases surgery can make glasses unnecessary, especially if the correction needed is very weak. *But it is important to remember that it is the accommodation needed for clear vision that causes the convergence and hence the esotropia.* Children with accommodative esotropia are farsighted. And that farsightedness is a refractive error of the eyes, not a problem in the eye muscles that can be corrected with surgery. Relying on surgery to do what should be done with glasses may risk an *outward* deviation of the eyes.

Some eye doctors occasionally recommend treating accommodative esotropia with eyedrops or ointments *(miotics)* instead of glasses. In part, the medication works by inducing accommodation locally, so the reflex that includes convergence and accommodation is not activated. The medications may not work as well as glasses, and they can have side effects (especially pupillary cysts) that limit their long-term usefulness. But they can be helpful, for example, during the summer months when glasses would interfere with swimming.

Although more than one type of treatment may be required and periodic follow-up is important, children with all forms of esotropia have an excellent chance of growing up with good vision and straight eyes. In many cases, they have useful binocular vision and may even have normal stereopsis.

9

Exotropia:
Eyes That Turn Out

A lex *was almost four years old when his parents first noticed his left eye drifted outward. He tended to close the eye whenever he was outside on a sunny day. Over the following few months the closing got worse, to the point that his older brother started calling him Popeye. At first the eye drifted outward only occasionally, and just for a moment. But gradually the deviation became more frequent. It began to happen both outdoors and indoors, and the eye stayed out for longer periods of time.*

❧

Alex has exotropia—sometimes called "wall eyes"—the condition in which one eye turns out. It is not common, but in any group of several hundred otherwise normal children there will probably be at least one with exotropia. Like accommodative esotropia, exotropia usually starts between the ages of 2 and 5 and is frequently first seen

LEFT EXOTROPIA. The right eye is looking at the camera, but the left eye is turned outward. The deviation, which measures about 20 degrees by the Hirshberg method, is likely intermittent, at least initially. Typically, the eyes are better aligned when looking at near than at distant objects.

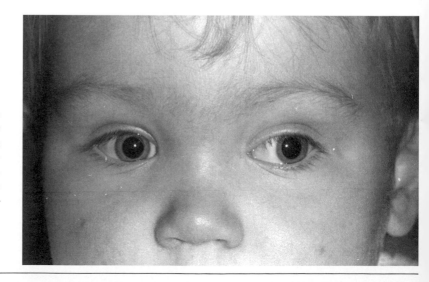

In its early stages, the deviation lasts only a few seconds and goes away with a blink or a change of gaze.

when the child is tired or sick. It rarely starts before 6 months of age.

In the typical childhood-onset exotropia, one eye (or alternate eyes) turns outward briefly and intermittently when the child looks at something 10 or more feet away. Parents may have difficulty seeing the deviation in its early stages. It lasts only a few seconds and goes away with a blink or a change of gaze. What usually happens is that as the parent approaches to look at the child more closely, the child looks at the parent and the eyes straighten.

Over time—sometimes weeks, sometimes months—one eye or the other will start turning out more often and more easily, but only when the child is looking across the room or farther. The deviation usually progresses, either in degree or, more typically, in the frequency and the duration of each occurrence.

It would be nice if we knew the cause, but unfortunately we don't. Children with exotropia have normal refractive errors; their need for glasses is no different from that of children with no strabismus. One might reason that, if hyperopia (farsightedness) causes esotropia and exotropia is the opposite of esotropia, then myopia (nearsightedness) must cause exotropia. This reasoning is logical but it is not supported by facts. Myopic children have no more exotropia than children who are not myopic. Like other forms of strabismus, exotropia can run in families. But the exact pattern of inheritance is unclear, and in many cases it occurs with no family history at all.

Double vision and suppression: Children who have one eye that turns out are very likely to see two images: that is, they see double. By blinking hard or rubbing one eye, they may restore the alignment and eliminate the double vision. If that doesn't work, they may close or cover the eye. Closing one eye outdoors, especially in the sunlight, is a common and typical sign of intermittent exotropia. Some children close one eye while watching television.

Gradually, children with exotropia may deal with their double vision by unconsciously suppressing the image from the deviating eye (in the same way as children with esotropia do). Once the second image is suppressed, they are not able to tell whether the eye is turned out or is aligned with the other. If amblyopia ("lazy eye") develops as a result, vision is usually not as poor as it may be in children with esotropia.

Gradually the deviation may become more constant. If one eye is turning out often and staying out when the child is looking far away, the eye may gradually start to turn out intermittently when the child is looking at something near. In time—perhaps months or even years—one eye might turn out constantly regardless of where the child is looking.

Treatment   If amblyopia has developed, it is treated first, with patching of the preferred eye. Sometimes the patch is alternated between the eyes—that is, patching one eye one day and the other the next.

The main treatment for exotropia is surgery. But before recommending surgery, some ophthalmologists may try nonsurgical treatments. These include minus lenses (glasses for myopia) even if the child is not myopic. Minus lenses will force the child's eyes to accommodate (and converge) to see clearly and can help to control exotropia. Exercises are helpful in one type of exotropia (convergence insufficiency). Unfortunately, exercises do not work as well for other forms of exotropia, or for other kinds of strabismus.

These nonsurgical treatments may delay surgery, but if one eye is turning out often and easily, surgery is generally indicated. The operation is usually performed when it is apparent to the family and the ophthalmologist that the deviation has progressed to the point that it can no longer be controlled (one eye turns out easily and stays there, not returning with the next blink or change of gaze), or if the child must close one eye to avoid double vision.

Convergence insufficiency   One form of exotropia, called convergence insufficiency, deserves special mention. Children with this problem have straight eyes when they look at something far away, but their eyes tend to turn out when they look at something up close—for example, when they're reading. The condition is aptly named; the eyes cannot converge as well as they should. As a result, these children may experience eyestrain when reading. The problem usually begins in the teens or young adulthood, so it's rarely the cause of poor reading in elementary school.

Treatment: Convergence insufficiency is treated with orthoptic exercises that can be done at home. "Pencil push-ups" are a time-honored and effective treatment. The patient holds a pencil at arm's length and focuses on the writing on the pencil. The pencil is then slowly brought closer, inducing accommodation and convergence, and is held at reading distance. Sometimes a light is used instead of a pencil. Hand-held prisms may be added to stimulate more convergence. The exercises are generally continued for a few months. Over time, the symptoms improve, though if they recur, exercises may need to be restarted.

Almost all cases of exotropia can be treated effectively. With consistent follow-up, glasses, patching, exercises, and surgery as needed, the prognosis for good vision and straight eyes is very good.

10 Less Common Forms of Strabismus

An eye can deviate not only horizontally, but vertically, so that it is higher or lower than the other eye. If the nonfixing eye is higher, the condition is called *hypertropia*; if lower it is called *hypotropia*.

Vertical deviations are more likely than horizontal deviations to be *incomitant*, or larger in one direction of gaze than another. Children with an incomitant deviation are often able to control the deviation by turning or tilting their head into a position that allows the eyes to be straight and avoids double vision. It is this abnormal and persistent head tilt that is often first noticed by the family. Sometimes they think something is wrong with the bones or muscles of the neck. The eye misalignment itself may be so slight that it cannot be easily seen.

There are several specific types of vertical strabismus. The first three listed, overaction of the inferior oblique, overaction of the superior oblique and dissociated vertical deviation, are much more common in children who have or have had congenital esotropia.

Overaction of the inferior oblique

When the inferior oblique muscle contracts, it pulls the eye up-and-in, so that it looks across the nose toward the opposite side of the fore-

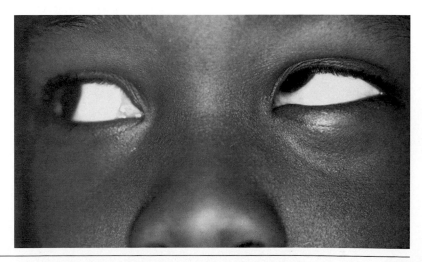

OVERACTION OF THE INFERIOR OBLIQUE. The left eye is turned up in right gaze by the excessive pull of the inferior oblique muscle.

head. When this muscle pulls too strongly, the overaction (usually in both eyes) is seen whenever the child looks to either side: the eye that is turned toward the nose is too high. In other words, when the child looks to the left, the right eye is higher, and when the child looks to the right, the left eye is higher. Inferior oblique overaction is often associated with a V pattern *(see page 90)*. If the deviation is very noticeable, the muscle may need to be weakened surgically. If the problem is associated with a horizontal strabismus, both conditions can be corrected at the same time.

Overaction of the superior oblique

The superior oblique muscle pulls the eye down-and-in, to allow the right eye, for example, to look down and to the left. If it pulls too strongly, the eye that is turned to the nose is too low. As with overaction of the inferior oblique muscle, overaction of the superior oblique tends to occur in patients who also have horizontal strabismus. It often is associated with an A pattern *(see page 90)*.

Dissociated vertical deviation (DVD)

With DVD, one eye, or either eye alternately, slowly rises. The eye may remain in that position, or it may return to be level with the other eye after the child blinks or looks somewhere else. Most often the affected eye rises intermittently, but occasionally one eye is constantly higher. Sometimes an eye rises only when it is covered.

Unlike overaction of both the inferior and superior oblique muscles, which are visible only when the eyes look to the side, DVD is often present in all gazes, including straight ahead. It may exist alone or in combination with any other type of strabismus.

DVD has a very characteristic pattern on cover testing. In other forms of vertical strabismus, fixation with the higher eye makes the other turn downward behind the cover. In DVD, the other eye either stays straight or actually rises behind the cover. It is this paradoxical, see-saw dissociation of the eyes that gives DVD its name.

If one eye is noticeably higher than the other and the deviation occurs frequently, surgical correction may be warranted.

Superior oblique palsy

In congenital superior oblique palsy, this muscle is weak from birth. The condition occurs fairly frequently, perhaps once in every several thousand otherwise healthy children.

The nerves to the eye muscles arise from the brainstem. For some unknown reason the trochlear nerve (4th cranial nerve), which supplies the superior oblique muscle, does not function properly,

DISSOCIATED VERTICAL DEVIATION.

Top: The eyes are well aligned.

Center: With a cover over the left eye, that eye begins to dissociate, drifting upward (left). The left eye is now hypertropic, even without the cover (right). The deviation can also occur during periods of visual inattention or when the child is tired.

Bottom: The right eye begins to dissociate upward behind the cover (left). There is now a right hypertropia without the cover (right).

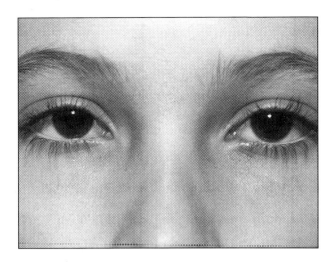

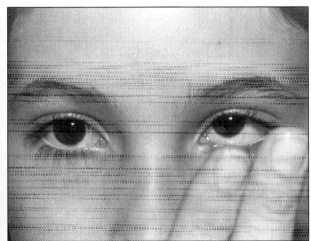

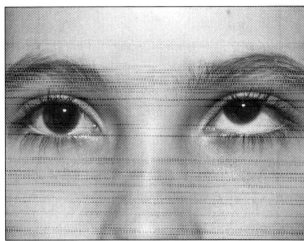

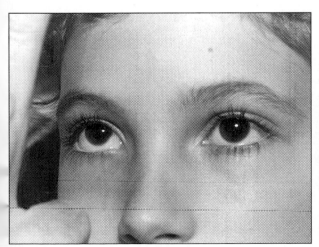

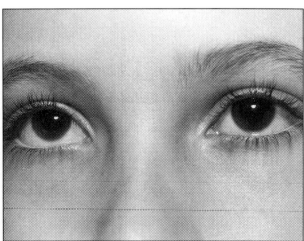

LEFT SUPERIOR OBLIQUE PALSY

The eyes are aligned in the straight ahead position. In more severe cases, the head must be tilted for the eyes to be level.

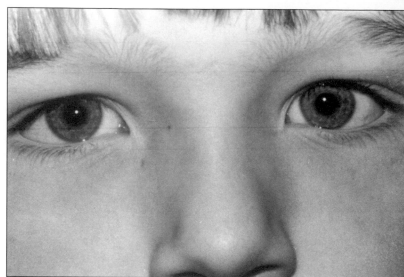

On gaze to the right and down, the left eye depresses less because of the weakness of the left superior oblique.

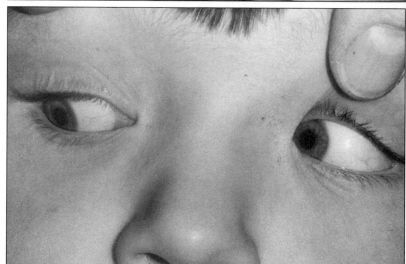

On gaze to the right and up, the left eye elevates more because the unopposed left inferior oblique overacts.

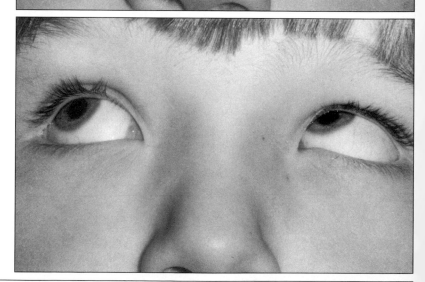

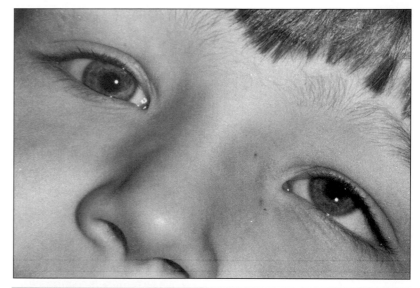

With the head tilted to the left shoulder, the left superior oblique cannot depress the eye, which therefore elevates more.

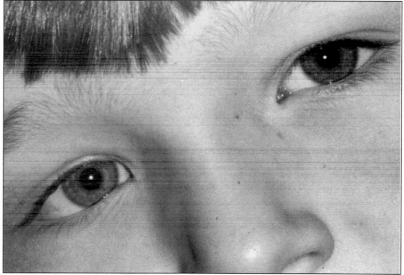

With the head tilted to the right shoulder, the eyes are aligned.

resulting in a partially or completely paralyzed muscle. It is unusual for other neurologic problems to be associated, especially in congenital or longstanding cases.

The normal function of the superior oblique muscle is to pull the eye down-and-in. When it is weak the affected eye is slightly higher than normal. But it is higher only in certain positions of gaze or in certain head positions. The worst deviation is characteristically on gaze to the opposite side and with the head tilted to the side of the higher eye. The eyes are usually level when the head is tilted to the side opposite the affected eye and the chin is lowered a bit.

Congenital superior oblique palsy is probably the most common ocular cause of an abnormal head position.

The treatment of vertical strabismus

In mild cases, no treatment may be needed. If the deviation or the head tilt is severe, surgery can adjust the pull of one or more eye muscles in order to make the eyes more level. Either the higher eye can be lowered or the lower eye can be raised. In either case, successful alignment of the eyes may allow the child to have a normal head position.

A and V patterns

As noted earlier, the deviating eye of a child with horizontal strabismus, whether esotropia or exotropia, usually maintains the same angle of deviation no matter which direction the child looks. If the angle of deviation is 10°, that angle will remain 10° regardless of the direction of gaze. That constancy of the angle of deviation is called *comitance*, and, as noted above, the deviations are called *comitant*.

Although *incomitance* is more typical of vertical deviations, some horizontal deviations are incomitant as well. As the child looks up or down, the angle of the deviation changes.

Let's assume a child has an esotropia of 5° on looking up, 10° in straight-ahead gaze, and 15° on looking down. If the positions of the eyes from up-gaze to down-gaze could be marked on the face, a line connecting them would look like the letter V. The term *V syndrome (or V pattern)* describes this pattern. It can occur with either esotropia or exotropia. A V pattern exotropia is worst on upgaze

The opposite pattern, which can also exist with either esotropia or exotropia, is called *A syndrome* (or *A pattern*). Suppose one eye turns out 5° on looking up, 10° in straight-ahead gaze, and 15° on looking down. A line connecting these positions would look like the letter A.

V PATTERN STRABISMUS. In upgaze the eyes diverge more. In downgaze the eyes converge more. Note the resemblance to the letter V, whether the underlying deviation is esotropia or exotropia. Inferior oblique muscle overaction is often present in at least one eye.

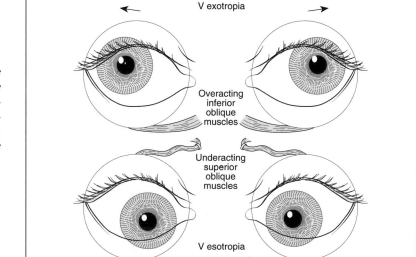

V exotropia

Overacting inferior oblique muscles

Underacting superior oblique muscles

V esotropia

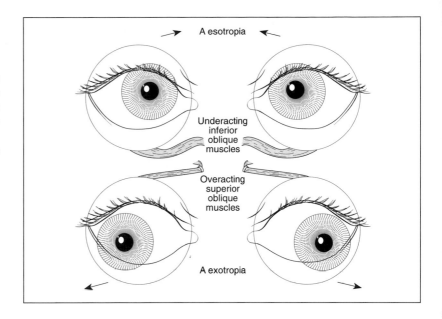

A PATTERN STRABISMUS. In upgaze the eyes converge more. In downgaze the eyes diverge more. Note the resemblance to the letter A, whether the underlying deviation is esotropia or exotropia. Superior oblique muscle overaction is often present in at least one eye.

An A pattern esotropia is worst on upgaze.

Usually V patterns are present with overaction of both inferior oblique muscles and A patterns with overaction of both superior oblique muscles. The inferior obliques abduct the eyes most on upgaze and the superior obliques abduct on downgaze. But sometimes there is no such overaction.

Occasionally, an A or V pattern will cause an abnormal head position. If, for example, a horizontal strabismus in straight-ahead gaze goes away when the child looks up or down, that child will very likely tilt the chin down or up into a position where the eyes are aligned.

When possible, an A or V syndrome is treated surgically at the same time that the primary problem, the esotropia or exotropia, is corrected.

Duane's syndrome

Duane's syndrome is an unusual type of strabismus. Children who have it have limited eye movements. In the most common form one eye will not move to the side. The eyes are aligned in straight-ahead gaze, but when the child looks to the side of the affected eye it will not move. Less commonly the limitation of movement is toward the nose. In the least common form the affected eye will move very little horizontally in either direction.

In any of these types the affected eye may also move up or down when the child is looking in toward the nose. This upshoot or downshoot, as it is called, can be dramatic and unsightly. Often the eyelids close slightly when the child looks toward the nose and the eye

DUANE'S SYNDROME.

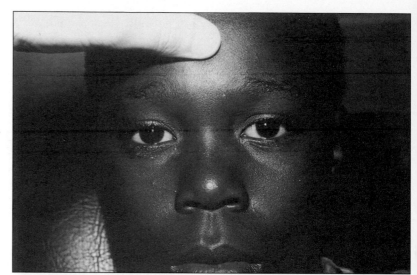

The eyes are aligned when the child looks straight ahead.

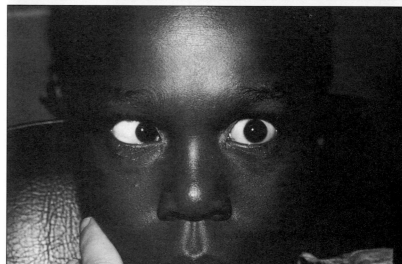

On left gaze, the left eye does not abduct well.

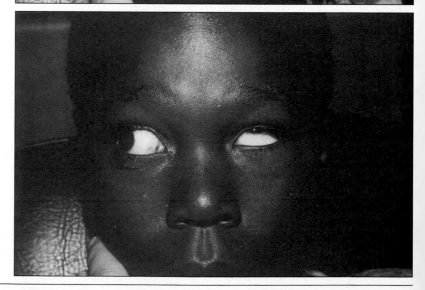

On right gaze, the left eye upshoots.
(photos courtesy Ed Wilson, MD)

will actually retract slightly back into the orbit.

Duane's syndrome is a congenital defect of unknown cause that usually occurs in otherwise healthy children, a bit more often in girls than in boys and more often in the left eye than in the right. It nearly always affects only one eye, but it may be bilateral. It was first described by Dr. Alexander Duane of New York at the turn of the centery.

A little more is known about the cause of Duane's syndrome than that of many of the other types of strabismus. Normally, nerves from the brainstem connect to each of the muscles that move the eye. In a child with Duane's syndrome, the electrical signals are transmitted appropriately, but not to the correct muscles. As a result the affected eye is out of alignment with the normal eye, which is getting the correct signals to the correct muscles.

Duane's syndrome can be quite confusing to parents. If the left eye does not move to the left on attempted gaze to that side (it remains pointed straight ahead) and the right eye does move, the parents may think the right eye is abnormal.

Most children with Duane's syndrome have no face turn because the eyes are aligned on looking straight ahead. But in some affected children the eyes are aligned only on looking to one side, so these children will turn their face to that position. If the compensatory face turn is noticeable, surgery can move the affected eye so the child can view the environment without a face turn, but the limitation of eye movement will remain. Fortunately, most patients do not require surgery since their eyes are aligned in the straight-ahead position.

Brown's syndrome

In the 1950s Dr. Harold Brown, also of New York, described a condition that was new to ophthalmologists at that time: a syndrome in which one eye cannot look up-and-in. The problem is a too-tight superior oblique muscle that cannot relax, resulting in an eye that is unable to elevate normally.

This condition usually exists from birth, but it may also be acquired, sometimes following an injury or an inflammation around the trochlea, and sometimes for no apparent reason. Parents notice that when their child looks up, one eye rises more than the other. Often they think that the higher eye that is the abnormal one, but actually it is the lower eye that is abnormal. The condition is usually associated with a V pattern exotropia. Rarely, it is bilateral.

Brown's syndrome occurs with varying degrees of involvement. To use both eyes together, a child with severe limitation assumes an abnormal head position, usually with the chin up and the face turned away from the affected eye (in an attempt to look down-and-out, away from the position in which there is a limitation of movement). Surgery

BROWN'S SYNDROME

When looking up and to the left, the right eye does not elevate normally.

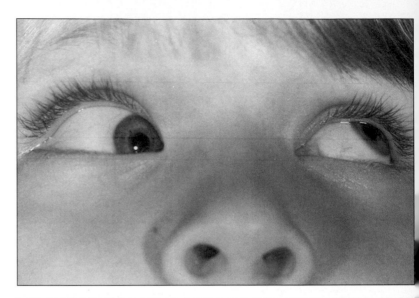

Its elevation improves when looking up and to the right.

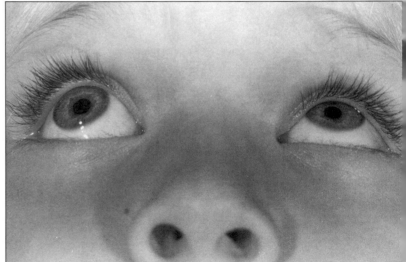

may be suggested to eliminate the abnormal compensatory head position. Fortunately, most cases of Brown's syndrome are so mild that surgery is not required.

There are also less common forms of strabismus. Some occur in conjunction with various diseases or as a result of trauma or surgery. Almost all of them can be improved with treatment. Sometimes the outcome is not ideal, but nearly all patients with strabismus can be helped to keep their deviation controlled enough for it to be hard for others to notice.

11   Amblyopia

Matt's failure on the kindergarten vision screening test had been totally unexpected. His parents were sure he could see just fine; he could find the smallest specks on the floor and the farthest planes in the sky. The pediatrician's nurse had tested his eyesight just one year before and found it normal.

On the recommendation of the pediatrician, Matt's parents took him to an eye doctor. Sure enough, Matt had a problem—his left eye was legally blind. The doctor told Matt's parents that he had amblyopia, which people often call "lazy eye." His right eye was fine; that's why no one suspected that anything was wrong. The doctor prescribed glasses, but the vision in Matt's left eye was still poor.

Amblyopia is defined as poor vision in an otherwise normal eye that begins in childhood. So how had Matt passed the eye test the year before? In all likelihood, he had peeked with his right eye. He hadn't meant to cheat; he was just trying to do what the nurse had asked, to name the figures on the chart.

Both of Matt's eyes were straight. It would have been better if his left eye had crossed. Then his problem would have been recognized and he would have been treated sooner. There is an old saying about amblyopia: "The doctor sees nothing and the patient sees little." In other words, amblyopic eyes typically look as if they should see well. But the condition can cause a lifetime of poor vision.

Amblyopia is the most common reason for children to have less-than-normal corrected vision. The disorder is so common, in fact, that it accounts for more cases of vision impairment than all other causes combined (as many as 3%, or 9 million, Americans are affected). It occurs more often in children who have close relatives with amblyopia, and almost always affects only one eye.

Amblyopia begins during the first few years of life, when vision is developing. For some reason the child prefers the other eye, so the affected eye does not develop normal vision. The visual acuity of an amblyopic eye can range from nearly normal to worse than 20/400, and it cannot be corrected with glasses. With early treatment, however, the chance that a child will recover vision is very good.

The visual acuity of an amblyopic eye can range from nearly normal to worse than 20/400, and it cannot be corrected with glasses.

Types of amblyopia

All children with amblyopia have had some kind of abnormal visual experience during the first years of life. The nature of that experience determines the type of amblyopia.

Strabismic amblyopia   The most common type of amblyopia is called strabismic because it affects a deviated eye. Vision in that eye is unconsciously suppressed to prevent double vision. It does not matter whether the eye turns inward, outward, or vertically, deviates markedly, or drifts only slightly.

Not all children with strabismus develop amblyopia. Some, for example, alternate the use of their eyes, in a way exercising each, so that amblyopia does not have the opportunity to develop.

Deprivation amblyopia   This type of amblyopia is the most severe. It develops when a young child's eyes are deprived of normal visual experience by some condition that prevents light from reaching the retina.

Cataracts are the most common cause. Infants whose corneas are clouded at birth or who have other opacities in their eyes, or eyelid growths that cover the pupil and are left untreated for many months, may also develop deprivation amblyopia. (Mild partial cataracts, especially in older children, and ptosis [droopy eyelids] that only partly close the eye will normally not cause an eye to become amblyopic.)

Urgent treatment may be needed. A dense cataract, for example, should be removed even in the first days of life. Delay could result in extremely poor vision despite successful surgery. (After the cataract is removed, optical correction must be provided in the form of glasses, contact lenses or intraocular lenses.)

Anisometropic amblyopia   The most difficult amblyopia to detect is anisometropic amblyopia, a condition in which the eyes have different refractive errors, making one eye out-of-focus compared to the other. Whether that eye is nearsighted, farsighted, or astigmatic, it is not used and so it fails to develop good vision. This is the kind of amblyopia Matt had.

No one, not the parents, the family doctor, nor the pediatrician, has any reason to suspect a problem when the eyes are perfectly straight and the good eye sees normally. So the amblyopia typically remains undiscovered and treatment is delayed until the child has a vision screening test. As in Matt's case, this often happens in kindergarten.

Bilateral amblyopia   Amblyopia usually affects only one eye. But there are a few conditions that can cause bilateral amblyopia.

Bilateral cataracts and similar conditions can block light from reaching both retinas. Another cause is a strong refractive error in both eyes. This type (*isoametropic amblyopia*) is especially likely to develop when the refractive error remains uncorrected until late in childhood. Like its one-eyed cousin, anisometropic amblyopia (*above*), isoametropic amblyopia is treated with optical correction as early as possible. Patching is not usually needed. In most cases the vision gradually gets better when the child wears the proper glasses, but sometimes it doesn't improve to 20/20.

Treatment

For all types of amblyopia, early treatment is best. Vision scientists believe the parts of the visual system that are defective in amblyopic children are actually in the brain. Faced with continued suppression, visual deprivation or unfocused images, the brain cells connected to the amblyopic eye (or eyes) gradually stop working. Once this happens, it may become impossible to reverse amblyopia.

Deprivation amblyopia from a dense cataract, for example, tends to become permanent by several months of age. On the other hand, depending on the kind of abnormal visual experience and how bad it was, amblyopia treatment may be effective even years after its onset. A few children with anisometropic amblyopia can be improved as late as 12 years of age. Strabismic amblyopia may even be reversible in adults who have lost the use of their good eye.

Prescribing glasses or surgically removing a cataract is sometimes the only treatment required. Unfortunately, surgery to align a strabismic eye cannot make it see better.

For most children, it is necessary to cover the normal eye with a patch or similar device in order to force the child to use the weak eye and strengthen its vision. If glasses are prescribed for the amblyopic eye, they are worn with the patch. Patching should be prescribed by an eye doctor, and its effects should be monitored at regular intervals.

Keeping the patch in place: Often children object to patching and try their best to get the patch off or to peek around it, especially at

Vision scientists believe the parts of the visual system that are defective in amblyopic children are actually in the brain.

All children wearing an eye patch need to be monitored by an eye doctor at regular intervals. The patch prevents light from reaching the retina and too much patching may cause an amblyopia in the good eye.

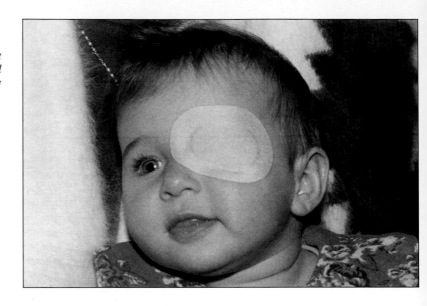

PATCHING FOR AMBLYOPIA. If the right eye is amblyopic, forcing a young child to use that eye will almost certainly improve its vision.

first. Remember, the patch forces the child to use the "bad" eye, and it may be pretty bad indeed until the treatment starts to work. There is no easy solution to this problem. Distraction tends to work best for infants and toddlers, especially when the patch is first applied. Lots of attention, play, hugging and support will be required until the child gets used to the patch and begins to see better. Bribery is effective with toddlers, and older children may be persuaded to listen to reason.

Some parents are more successful maintaining occlusion by using a device that fits onto the glasses and prevents the child from peeking with the good eye. Elbow restraints are useful for really resistant children. The inflatable cuffs that are used for swimming can work just as well if they are positioned across the elbows. In some cases, cycloplegic eyedrops or defocused glasses can blur the "good" eye, taking the place of a patch. This approach is called "penalization" of the dominant eye.

If all else fails, parents may have to stop the patching for several weeks or months, then try again. Perhaps by then they will have increased their resolve to be firm. Or perhaps the child will be in a new stage of development and will be less resistant.

Avoiding irritation from the patch: Some children experience skin irritation from the adhesive patch. This is rarely due to an allergy, but if it is, a different brand of patch should solve the problem. More often the irritation is the result of moisture from perspiration, and abrasion of the skin every time the tape is pulled off. Attaching the occluder to the glasses is one solution to this problem. Another useful trick is to apply tincture of benzoin or Skin Prep® to the skin. This forms a protective coating, so the tape sticks to the coating rather than to the tender skin around the eye. (It's important to keep the skin preparations away from the eye itself.) Both products are available from pharmacies without a prescription.

Length of time required: Patching usually begins on a nearly full-time basis. Many pediatric ophthalmologists prefer to allow a brief "time off" each day to reduce the possibility that too much patching will cause amblyopia in the good eye. Certainly it's not necessary to patch the eye when the child is asleep, though some parents find it easier just to leave the patch on, especially through naps.

Vision is then re-assessed after a period of time determined by the age of the child. Generally the eye doctor will schedule a follow-up visit at a frequency of 1 week for every year of age—that's every 3 days for a child of 6 months, but every 2 months for a child who is 8 years old. (The visit intervals can be lengthened when patching is performed part-time.) The advantage of early patching is obvious: not only is it more effective, it works more quickly as well.

Intensive patching is continued until the amblyopic eye becomes as good as the other eye or until it stops improving. Children with strabismus may start to cross the eye that had been the straight one. Many parents find this alarming, but they can actually be pleased to see this change. It means that the child is able, for the first time, to use either eye. (Occasionally it may be necessary to switch the patch to the other eye.)

Results: The goal for every child is to achieve the best possible vision in each eye. In mild cases, 20/20 vision is often possible. In more severe cases, a plateau is reached and then there is no further improvement.

In about half the children treated, the improved vision will remain stable without patching. They will need only occasional re-checks. The other half will "slip"; their amblyopia will recur, but usually to a lesser degree than before. They will need patching again, either full- or part-time, until the lost vision is regained.

All children should be followed until they are about 9 years old. After that age, the vision in the amblyopic eye tends to remain stable, even if the child uses the good eye all the time.

When treatment doesn't work   Some cases of amblyopia are resistant to treatment. Perhaps there is something structurally defective in the eye. Children who have severe physical or developmental problems should perhaps not even start treatment, or should have only a brief therapeutic trial.

Parents must always remember that, although vision is important, we must consider the whole child, not just an eye. The decision to stop treatment can be difficult, but it is sometimes best for both the child and the family. For children with useful vision in only one eye, safety glasses and sports goggles are prescribed to protect that eye. As long as the eye remains healthy, such children see normally in almost every respect.

≈⁀

Certainly by age 5, and ideally by age 3 or 4, all children should have their vision measured, separately in each eye, by their primary care provider. When amblyopia is found in younger children, the treatment can be dramatically successful. It is not unusual for a 2-year-old who is legally blind from strabismic amblyopia to achieve completely normal vision in less than a month.

The challenge is to find very young children with amblyopia who don't have strabismus. Some of the most exciting research in pediatric ophthalmology involves screening of large populations for amblyopia. One method involves photographing the pupils of infants and toddlers. Perhaps such photorefractions, which may uncover amblyogenic factors early, will prevent stories like Matt's from being repeated so often in the future.

12 Eye Muscle Surgery

Erin, not yet two years old, had been through a lot since her right eye started to cross. First, her left eye was patched. That did not help the crossing, and in fact it made the left eye start to turn in. Then she was given glasses. They seemed to help some, but the crossing was still pretty obvious. So the doctor recommended surgery on her eye muscles.

Erin's parents were concerned about the surgery and had many questions. Her mom had heard that the eyes had to be taken out for this kind of operation, and that made both parents particularly nervous.

The surgery recommended for Erin is typical of most eye muscle operations. It is designed to straighten the eyes by changing the way the muscles pull. The effect is often dramatic *(see photos on page 108).* Erin's transformation took only about an hour, and she went home from the hospital two hours later.

It's very rare for strabismus to be so severe that surgery cannot correct it. And there's no truth to the claim that it can be "too late" for surgery. One charming lady we know finally had her operation at age 86.

The benefits of surgery

Normal appearance and self-esteem   "But isn't the surgery just cosmetic?" parents often ask. This question brings to mind the movie star who doesn't like the shape of his nose or the size of her breasts—people who want to improve parts of their bodies that are already normal. But it's simply not normal to have one's eyes looking in different directions. It's been that way since ancient times, when cross-eyed figures were used to represent evil spirits.

People who have strabismus are seldom allowed to forget about it, especially if the deviation is severe. School-age children may be teased mercilessly. Adolescents suffer self-image problems as they begin to be interested in the opposite sex. Adults may find that their careers are adversely affected, especially if their work involves contact with the public.

Cross-eyed people are reminded of their disfigurement every time they make eye contact with someone who doesn't know which eye to look at. The 86-year-old lady mentioned above is a good example. She had had a successful operation as a child, but over time, as often happens, her eye had again drifted out of alignment. She became so self-conscious that she was embarrassed to go to the grocery store.

Improved function Eye muscle surgery can improve the visual function of some patients. Older children (or adults) with recently acquired strabismus may have double vision and lose depth perception. These symptoms can be troublesome. For example, if Tommy is playing baseball, he won't know which ball to hit.

For children whose strabismus is incomitant (*see Chapter 10*), turning or tilting their head is the only way they can use their eyes together. (In rare cases, the eye muscles are so tightly pulled out of position that one eye cannot be centered and its vision is impaired.) Similarly, many children with nystagmus (involuntary eye movements) can control their problem and achieve better vision only by holding their head to one side. Their head positions become nearly constant, and make them look and feel different from their peers. Eye muscle surgery may permit all of these children to resume normal posture.

Surgery like Erin's helps the two eyes work together to make one image. Exactly how well depends on the individual.

What surgery can and cannot do

Vision: One thing Erin's surgery will not do is to make her see more clearly. That has already been accomplished by patching and glasses. In rare cases, a child whose glasses have failed to control the eye crossing will need weaker glasses, or none at all, after surgery. But that is the exception. It's best to assume that straightening a crooked eye will not improve its vision or change its need for glasses.

Stereopsis: Even the most accurate surgery can't restore perfect stereoscopic vision unless the visual areas of the brain have the potential to develop this kind of visual coordination. The best results are expected in patients whose strabismus begins after the first few years of life, remains intermittent, and is accurately repaired soon after it begins.

Will Erin's eyes work together perfectly to make a stereoscopic image after surgery? Probably not. But this actually isn't such a terrible problem. After all, most children with strabismus seem to function normally in most visual tasks.

Most specialists believe that if the two eyes work together, even partially, they are more likely to remain straight or nearly straight after surgery. For a constant deviation in infants, the best chance for the eyes to work together is with early surgery, within the first 2 years of life. For intermittent deviations and those acquired after infancy, the timing of surgery should be individualized, depending on their severity and symptoms.

Alignment: It would be nice if the surgeon could tell Erin's parents that her surgery will work perfectly, that her eyes will be perfectly aligned when she wakes up and will remain so for the rest of her life. In fact, however, it is usually not that way. In time, there will probably be at least a small amount of crossing or drifting in some direction. But this crossing is often hard to see. And if one has to look critically to detect it, it probably doesn't require more surgery.

Perhaps it's best, since strabismus seems so hard to "cure" completely, to consider Erin's problem as a condition to be "controlled." In about 80% of all cases, surgery can control strabismus so well that it's hard to see two months later. If not, or if it slips out of control later, it can almost always be improved with another operation.

The risks of surgery

In addition to its being reasonably effective, Erin's surgery is relatively safe. It's rare for the eyes to end up out of alignment in some way that can't be put right later. Complications affecting the vision could occur—for example, the retina could be damaged or a serious infection could set in—but these problems are extremely rare. Double vision occasionally happens after surgery, especially in patients age 7 or older, so that's one more reason it's better to operate early. However, double vision is rarely a serious problem (even in adults), and it can almost always be fixed. Other minor complications, such as wound irregularities or changes in eyelid position, sometimes occur but they are unusual.

Anesthesia problems, potentially disastrous, are exceptional in modern operating rooms. Erin's parents can help avoid problems by letting the surgeon know if she becomes ill just before surgery. Eye muscle surgery is elective; nothing terrible would happen if it had to be delayed several days or weeks. Some doctors worry that even a cold or earache may increase the chance of a complication from the anesthesia. For safety's sake it is better to reschedule surgery if the child is not in the best possible health.

What to expect

The actual experience of surgery is much less frightening today than it once was. Children hardly ever stay overnight in the hospital. They're more comfortable at home, they get more attentive care from their parents than from hospital personnel, and they're not surrounded by children who are sick and may even be infectious.

Before surgery   Several days before surgery, a nurse may show parents and older children the operating room and recovery room and explain what will happen step-by-step. As a precaution, a routine physical examination is usually performed (blood and urine tests may not be required). The risks of anesthesia increase if there is anything in the stomach when the child is put to sleep, so it's important to avoid solid food after midnight the night before surgery. Depending on the child's age, clear liquids may be permitted up to several hours before anesthesia is begun.

The surgery itself   On the day of surgery, Erin will be separated from her parents as little as possible. In many hospitals, her parents may be permitted to accompany her into the operating room, sitting with her as the anesthesia is breathed through a mask. Then the parent will be escorted to a waiting area. No needles are used until she is asleep, when the intravenous can be started painlessly.

It is not necessary to cut the skin. Incisions are made in the conjunctiva with scissors, not a scalpel or a laser. A small spring-loaded speculum holds the eyelids open, and a surgical assistant moves the eye from side to side as needed with forceps. Special hooks are used to hold the muscle that needs surgery.

Individual eye muscles will be weakened or strengthened during surgery, depending on the judgment of the surgeon and on whether the eye turns in, out, up or down. The most commonly performed procedure weakens the muscle by *recessing* it: moving the muscle's attachment to the sclera backward several millimeters.

In Erin's case, the medial rectus muscle pulls her eye too strongly toward her nose, so her surgeon will recess that muscle by cutting away connective tissue from the front and the sides of the muscle, putting a suture through it close to where it attaches to the eye, and

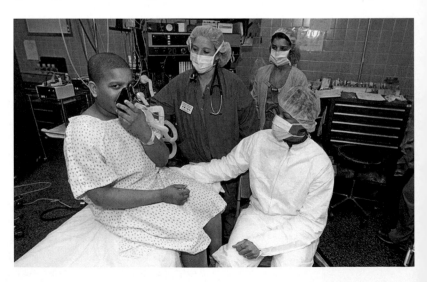

INDUCTION OF ANESTHESIA. The early phases of anesthesia are usually not unpleasant for the child. In this case, the mother's presence serves to calm his fears.

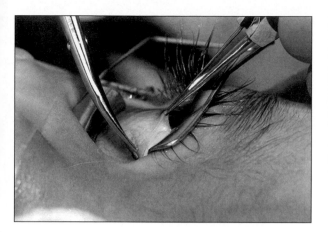

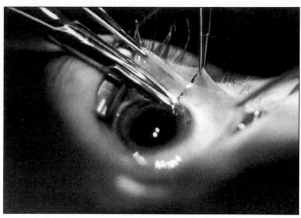

CONJUNCTIVAL INCISION IN MUSCLE SURGERY. (left). The eye is pulled up so that the scissors can be used to cut the conjunctiva in the inferonasal quadrant, so the medial rectus muscle can then be approached.

CLOSING THE CONJUNCTIVA (right). T.he conjunctival incision is closed with absorbable sutures at the completion of the surgery.

cutting the muscle just in front of the suture. The surgeon will then place sutures in the sclera at a carefully measured point. When the sutures are tied in position, the operated muscle will still pull the eye, but not so hard that the eye is crossed.

Strengthening operations, called *resections*, usually involve removing a measured length of muscle, then tightening the muscle much as a belt is tightened by moving its position in the buckle. In some cases a resection of one muscle (e.g., the left lateral rectus), is performed in conjunction with a recession of the opposite muscle (e.g., the left medial rectus).

For teenagers (and adults) an adjustable suture may be used with recessions or resections. This technique can be especially helpful in situations that involve more unpredictability—for example, in reoperations. The suture that attaches the muscle to the sclera has a slip knot that holds the muscle. When the patient wakes up or the local anesthesia has worn off, the knot is untied and the muscle is repositioned with minimal discomfort. This technique can't be used for children who are too young to cooperate for the adjustment.

Parents often ask, "How do you know how much to weaken or strengthen the muscle?" Surgeons refer to a table of specific amounts for different angles of deviation. Then they individualize this number based on their own experience, on the patient's measurements, and on other clinical data. The planning of eye muscle surgery demands as much skill as the surgery itself.

Sometimes a surgeon elects to operate on the non-deviating eye. When one eye is higher than the other, for example, the eyes can be made level either by raising the lower one or by lowering the higher one. The same logic applies when one eye turns in or out. It is especially important to include surgery on the "straight" eye if the angle is large or if there is an abnormal head posture.

At the end of the procedure, the incision is sewn together with tiny sutures that are hard to feel or see. These are absorbed after several days.

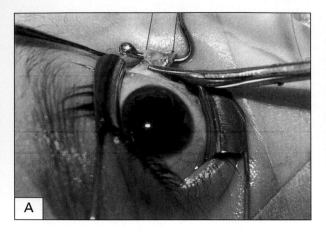

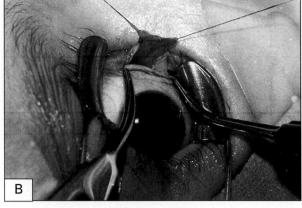

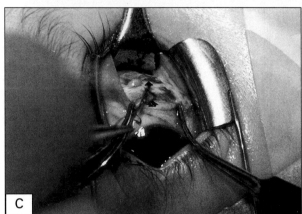

MUSCLE SURGERY—RECESSION. (A) In this surgery for esotropia, the medial rectus muscle is being detached from its original insertion. Absorbable sutures have been preplaced posterior to the scissors so the muscle cannot retract into the orbit. (B) The medial rectus has now been detached and the forceps grasp its original insertion. (C) The preplaced sutures have been sewn into the sclera so that the new insertion (small arrow) is several millimeters posterior to the old one (large arrow). The medial rectus will now adduct the eye less forcibly, decreasing the esotropia.

No blood products are transfused during the operation. *Some parents need to be reassured that the eye is never removed from the head.*

Recovery   Erin's surgery will take an hour or so. (Some types of eye muscle surgery are completed more quickly; complicated reoperations and procedures involving many muscles may take even longer.) Much of the time will be spent getting Erin safely to sleep and, after surgery, waking her up again. Erin will probably begin to stir in the operating room once the anesthesiologist stops administering the anesthesia. She will then be taken to the recovery room, where nurses will monitor her as the anesthesia wears off. Her parents will be at her bedside before she is fully awake.

At first Erin will be fretful, in and out of sleep and crying when she is awake. Her eyes will be sore, and the conjunctiva will be very red. The eyes will not be covered after surgery. Therefore, the parents will probably see a scant amount of blood in the tears. This is normal and is nothing for them to be frightened of. They will be instructed simply to wipe the blood away with a clean tissue or washcloth.

Erin will be ready to go home several hours after her surgery. Because the digestive system is affected by the anesthesia, it may take

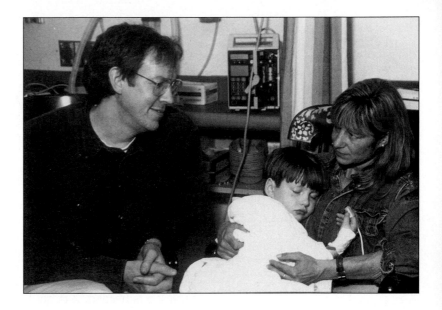

MUSCLE SURGERY — POST OPERATIVE. Generally children sleep for an hour or two after surgery. In this case, the parents comfort their son in the recovery room.

time before she can tolerate solid food. Water, chipped ice, and apple juice tend to be well tolerated. Her discomfort can be eased by any children's strength painkiller and a compress of cool or warm water. Hugs from Mom or Dad in a rocking chair will probably be even better.

By the next day the oozing and tearing will stop and Erin will probably be ready for a light breakfast. Her parents should discourage her from rubbing her eyes, but this is rarely a problem. Erin's activities will be restricted very little. It will be okay for her hair to be washed since she'll instinctively close her eyes, and she can even be given a shower. Her surgeon is likely to tell the parents that she should not go swimming or splash in the tub for a week or two.

Infections are quite rare. When one does occur, it's typically within the first week after surgery. The parents would notice the eye becoming more and more red, swollen, and uncomfortable.

Afterward   The effects of Erin's surgery will be seen as soon as she first opens her eyes. The alignment of her eyes is likely to change over time, though, especially during the healing period. After two weeks it should be hard to tell that surgery was done. (A slight irregularity of the conjunctiva may persist, though it is more likely after a complicated reoperation.) In about six weeks, her ophthalmologist will be able to tell how successful the surgery has been.

Routine checkups will be made at least every 6 to 12 months by her surgeon, who will have several goals in mind:

1. *Best possible vision in each eye.* Erin's glasses may need to be changed, or patching may be indicated. (If Erin hadn't had glasses, it might be necessary to prescribe them later.)

2. *Close-to-perfect alignment of the eyes.* Again, an adjusted (or

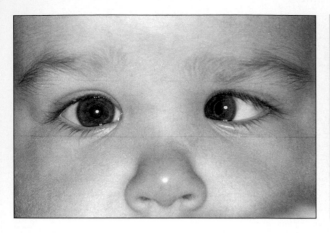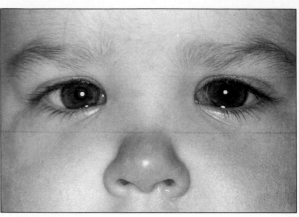

*THE EFFECT OF MUSCLE SURGERY .
Left: Preoperative photograph shows 20
degree left esotropia. Right: The same
child two days after both medial recti
were recessed.*

new) prescription may be given. Sometimes further surgery is needed.

3. *The fewest possible operations.* Usually when a second or third operation is needed, it is not because the first time was unsuccessful, but because the eyes have become misaligned after surgery. Even adults with a childhood history of strabismus may develop a deviation years later (this was the case with the 86-year-old lady mentioned at the beginning of this chapter).

The longer a child's eyes remain aligned after surgery, the better the chances of never needing another eye operation.

Injections as an alternative to surgery

During the past decade or so, some surgeons have developed an alternative treatment for strabismus that involves the injection of a drug into the eye muscles that need weakening. A minute dose of the drug, which has the brand name Botox, is injected directly into the eye muscle. Though this is the same compound that causes botulism, the injection causes no side effects like the dreaded disease, and can have very helpful weakening effects on the eye muscles.

The usefulness of Botox injections for strabismus is limited, though. The effect of the drug may be temporary, so about half of all patients need to be reinjected, and it is not particularly effective for large angles of misalignment.

Most surgeons prefer not to use this drug for young children, since injection may be difficult without anesthesia. But it may be helpful for older children (and adults) who have eye muscle palsies, such as after head trauma. (It is also used in treating other medical conditions—blepharospasm, for example— that have nothing to do with the eye muscles.)

MEDICAL
PROBLEMS

A NOTE TO PARENTS

In medical terminology, adding the suffix "-itis" means an inflammation of the part of the body represented by the root word. Conjunctivitis is an inflammation of the conjunctiva, which means that it is red, tender or swollen.

It is not necessarily infected, though it often is. When there is an infection, it can be passed on to someone else. That's why, in the story, Rebecca was sent home from school

"Steroids" is the shortened name for corticosteroids, which are substances produced naturally in the body by the adrenal glands, near the kidneys. Steroids are also medications that reduce inflammation and can help with the discomfort that comes with some forms of conjunctivitis. They do not usually affect the cause of the conjunctivitis; in fact, they might even mask its cause. You can recognize a steroid from the name. Compounds ending in "-one" (for example, hydrocortisone, prednisolone) usually contain a steroid.

Before using any medication in your child's eyes, read the label. Steroids should be used carefully and under the supervision of an ophthalmologist.

13 Conjunctivitis: The Pink Eye

Mrs. Fields had never given much thought to pink eye until she got a call from Rebecca's school. The school nurse asked her to pick up her daughter because she had pink eye. Rebecca had been fine at home that morning, but the nurse seemed adamant.

As Mrs. Fields drove to the school she began to wonder: Just what is pink eye, anyway? Is Rebecca in any danger? Could her sight be harmed? Is pink eye really that dangerous to the other children?

On the way home with Rebecca, she decided the nurse had overreacted. But later, when she looked closely at her daughter's right eye, she saw that it was in fact pink; some would even say red.

Mrs. Fields called her pediatrician, who asked a series of questions, most of which she answered in the negative: No, there is no problem with her vision; no, there's no sign of pain or discomfort; no, she's not light sensitive and she isn't closing her eye; no, there's no discharge. She had been sick with a cold for the past few days. The doctor told her to call back if there was any change and to come into the office if the redness didn't clear up in several days.

At one time or another nearly everyone has had conjunctivitis. Many of us probably got a couple of days off from school and maybe we even missed some days of work as adults. But common as it is, conjunctivitis is often confusing.

To understand conjunctivitis better, let's review the pertinent anatomy. The conjunctiva is the thin mucus membrane covering the front part of the eyeball (except the cornea) and the underside of the upper and lower lids. Normally the conjunctiva looks white, though it is actually translucent, like waxed paper. (The color comes from the underlying white sclera; on the backs of the lids, it looks slightly pink from the muscles beneath it.)

CONJUNCTIVITIS. The blood vessels are larger and more prominent and the back of the lid redder than normal.

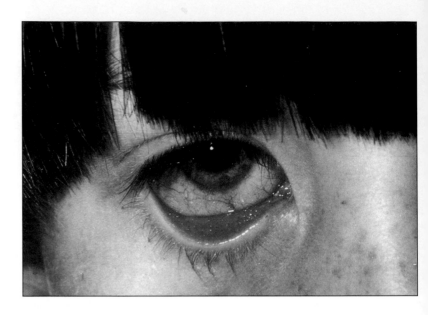

When the eye is irritated for any reason the conjunctival blood vessels become engorged, making the eyes look red. In rare cases *(hemorrhagic conjunctivitis)* a little blood might even leak out of the vessels into the conjunctiva.

Mucus and tear production

The irritation may also stimulate the production of a mucoid discharge, some of which tends to dry on the lashes. If the cause of the conjunctivitis is an infection, some of the moisture in the eye and some of the matter on the lashes will be pus, made up of white blood cells from the conjunctiva that have been killed by the infection.

Especially when the cornea is irritated, the conjunctiva and the lacrimal gland will respond by producing extra tears. These help to wash foreign material out of the eyes.

Conjunctivitis and colds

Tears normally drain from each eye into the *puncta*, the upper openings of the tear ducts. They are found at the edge of the upper and lower lids about a quarter of an inch from the inner corner of each eye. The tear ducts empty into the nose.

What does this have to do with conjunctivitis? Well, the tear ducts can also transmit bacteria and viruses from the nose upward, to infect the conjunctiva. So conjunctivitis is often associated with colds, though not always.

Colds and blocked tear ducts   When a child has a cold, there may be matter on the lashes, especially in the morning or after a nap. Inflammation from the respiratory infection causes swelling of the mucus membranes in the nose, blocking the lower opening of the tear duct. As a result, the mucus and tears normally produced by the conjunctiva can no longer drain into the nose. The eye may look wet, with a pool of tears visible along the lower lid. The tears evaporate, but the mucus tends to dry on the lids and lashes.

Blocked tear ducts alone do not cause the eyes to be red.

Children with blocked tear ducts almost always have more tearing and discharge when they have a cold. (Antibiotics, either oral or topical, may provide partial relief.) Very often, infants with blocked tear ducts are initially thought to have conjunctivitis. It is important to remember that blocked tear ducts alone do not cause the eyes to be red.

Determining the likely cause

Conjunctivitis may be caused by irritation, injury, infection or allergy. In many cases, the cause can be determined from a careful history.

Irritation   Mild conjunctivitis is most often caused by minor irritation. Smoke or dust in the air, chlorine in the swimming pool, and salt in sea water are common offenders. Our eyes may get red when we stay up late reading because we're too tired to blink often enough for tears to resurface the cornea. Dry air adds to the problem, giving the name to those all-night "red eye" airplane flights. Too much sun can result in ultraviolet damage to the conjunctiva and cornea, which causes *actinic conjunctivitis*; this is analagous to sunburn of the skin. Overwear and other sources of irritation from contact lenses are particularly common.

Treatment: The most effective treatment is to remove the source of irritation, use a tear substitute ("artificial tears") if necessary, and rest the eyes. They should get better in a matter of hours.,

Foreign body or injury   If there is any indication that a foreign body is in the eye or that the eye has been scratched, the child should be seen promptly by a doctor. Suggestive symptoms include sudden onset, profuse tearing, light sensitivity, and closing the eye. If the child has suddenly come running to Mom with a red, painful, tearing eye, there is almost certainly a corneal foreign body or abrasion, if not a more severe injury. Irritation of the cornea, much more than the conjunctiva, causes pain and light sensitivity.

Treatment: Unless it is apparent that the problem is minor, an ophthalmologist should be consulted. Fluorescein strips can be very helpful; the orange dye will outline a corneal abrasion or foreign body when a Wood's lamp or a blue light is directed at the eye.

Treatment of superficial injuries is discussed in more detail in Chapter 19. The key is to remove the foreign body (if there is one), apply an antibiotic ointment or drop, and perhaps patch the eye closed for a day or so. The eye should heal within a day or two.

Infection: viral   The typical infection is from a virus, which often causes an upper respiratory infection at the same time. *Adenovirus* is probably the most common organism. There are two classic forms: epidemic keratoconjunctivitis (EKC) and pharyngoconjunctival fever (PCF).

Epidemic keratoconjunctivitis is caused by adenovirus types 3, 8 and 19. Famous for its propensity to spread from one eye to the other and from person to person, this is a particularly severe infection. It typically begins with foreign body sensation, pain and redness and often causes inflammation of the lymph nodes in front of the ear. It also can involve the cornea. The infection may last as long as a month or more. As severe as it is symptomatically, it hardly ever causes permanent damage or threaten the eyesight.

Pharyngoconjunctival fever is caused by adenovirus type 3. This is similar to EKC but milder and associated with upper respiratory infection. There may be conjunctival hemorrhages. Cool compresses and tear substitutes are given as supportive treatment for both forms.

Herpes simplex conjunctivitis typically occurs at the same time as the primary infection with this virus. Usually, type 1 is the culprit, though a similar picture can be caused by type 2 herpes, and either can be acquired at birth. There may be an associated "cold sore" on or near the lids. In most cases, the primary infection is harmless and the cornea is not involved. But recurrent infections, which can develop years later, cause a characteristic infection called a *dendritic ulcer*, which can permanently damage the cornea. Topical treatment with trifluorothymidine, vidarabine, or idoxuridine may be required. An alternative is to debride the infected portion of the cornea.

Many other viruses can cause conjunctivitis as part of systemic infections. Included are Epstein-Barr (infectious mononucleosis), influenza type A, B or C, mumps, rubeola, and varicella zoster. Complications from these infections are extremely rare and treatment is supportive.

Infection: bacterial   In children, bacterial conjunctivitis is more common than in adults and may be even more common than viral conjunctivitis. A wide range of bacteria can be responsible, most normally present on the skin and even in the eye. Conjunctivitis results when natural defenses are insufficient to prevent these bacteria from multiplying. The symptoms are similar to viral conjunctivitis and are usually mild since the cornea is typically not involved.

Staphylococcus aureus is one of the most common bacterial causes. It is known for causing marginal blepharitis, an infection around the base of the lashes. Some cases are also complicated by partly allergic reactions in the peripheral cornea (staphallergic marginal ulcers and phlyctenules). *Staph epidermidis* causes a milder but similar range of involvement. Staph infections are well treated by almost all topical antibiotics. Lid scrubs and, under the supervision of an ophthalmologist, topical steroids are occasionally needed.

Streptococcal infections are also common in children. *Pneumococcus* is a normal resident of the respiratory tract. Like strep viridans, it occasionally proliferates to cause clinical conjunctivitis. Strep pyogenes and pneumococcus both can involve deeper structures within the eye, but both are very treatable with topical and systemic antibiotics.

Hemophilus influenza conjunctivitis, like other infections caused by this organism, is usually seen in younger children, during the winter months, and in association with respiratory infections. It has become less common since immunization programs have become widespread. Rarely, intraocular structures can be involved. Most cases respond to topical chloramphenicol, but blood dyscrasias have been reported following even topical administration.

Other bacterial causes of conjunctivitis in children include *Moraxella* and gram-negative rods: *E. Coli, Pseudomonas, Neisseria,* and other Hemophilus species.

Treatment: Infections of the conjunctiva are on the surface of the eye. Unless there has been some kind of damage to the cornea, most cases are self-limited. They get better in several days, with or without treatment. You may want to use artificial tears or cool compresses on the lids to relieve discomfort.

Cultures are rarely required, at least at first. A non-toxic topical antibiotic (such as sulfacetamide, erythromycin, gentamycin, tobramycin, bacitracin, tetracycline or chloramphenicol) may be prescribed several times daily. These are manufactured alone and in combination with polymyxin, neomycin, or gramicidin. Polytrim® is one combination—polymyxin and trimethoprim—with broad coverage that is well tolerated by children because it doesn't sting. Topical quinolones, ciprofloxacin, oxfloxacin and norfloxacin, have all been effective and well tolerated. Avoid preparations containing steroids. When systemic antibiotic treatment is prescribed for an associated respiratory infection or otitis, topical antibiotics may be unnecessary.

If the conjunctivitis does not respond to treatment after a week or more, avoid adding or substituting more topical medications, many of which are toxic and can cause a truly confusing conjunctivitis. It may be best to discontinue treatment, re-examine the eye, obtain a culture or a consultation, and try to direct specific treatment at the offending organism. In very many cases either the original cause was not bacterial or the bacteria have been eliminated. The child may obtain relief once the toxic or allergic effects of the eyedrops have subsided.

Infectious conjunctivitis is contagious (via the tears), and it is likely to spread to the second eye or to other family members. Parents should wipe away discharge with a disposable tissue, closing the eye and wiping from the upper lid down so as not to contact the eye. Sharing towels, washcloths and bedclothes should be avoided. Even adenovirus cannot leap through the air to land in someone else's eye, but little hands can rub the infected eye and touch too close to another eye. Frequent hand washing can be helpful, especially after the parents put the medicine in or pick up a used tissue. (Indeed, health care providers with infectious conjunctivitis should avoid contact with patients' eyes until the infection is cleared.)

Conjunctivitis in the newborn

Until the end of the 19th century, gonorrheal conjunctivitis was a common cause of blindness in newborns. Entire hospital wards were devoted to the lavage of these infants' eyes. The infection presents during the first several days after birth with severe lid swelling and great quantities of pus discharging from the eyes. What makes it so dangerous is that the organism can readily penetrate the intact corneal barrier, causing first an ulcer and, in some cases, perforation of the eyeball. Diagnosis is made by identification of gram-negative intracellular diplococci on smears and cultures. Systemic and topical penicillin remains the antibiotic of choice, though resistant strains have been reported.

The use of silver nitrate eyedrops in the newborn period nearly eliminated this devastating infection in the developed world. This solution does have its drawbacks, however. The first is that it can irritate the eyes, causing a "chemical conjunctivitis" during the first day or two following administration. It clears rapidly without treatment.

The second drawback is that silver nitrate is not very effective at preventing a much more common cause of neonatal conjunctivitis, Chlamydia trachomatis. Like gonorrhea, this is spread by sexual contact and is passed to the infant during the transit through the birth canal. (Even women who have no symptoms of venereal disease harbor an average of five different organisms in the cervix, and postpartem cultures show an average of three organisms already present in the eyes.) Children born by Caesarian section are not immune, however, as hand-to-eye contact can also pass the infection from parents or caregivers.

Chlamydial conjunctivitis typically begins about a week after birth with discharge, redness, and swelling that are much milder than in gonorrhea. It hardly ever damages the vision and cannot penetrate into the eye. On the other hand, it may infect the lungs several weeks later. The diagnosis can be confirmed by cell cultures showing inclusion bodies or by immunoassay. Treatment must be designed to counter, not just the conjunctivitis, but also the parents' presumed venereal infection and the baby's potential pneumonitis. Systemic erythromycin is the antibiotic therapy most recommended. Tetracycline is preferred for adults, except nursing mothers. Topically, either drug is effective prophylaxis against this organism.

Allergic conjunctivitis

Children can have several forms of allergic conjunctivitis. A common characteristic is its tendency to cause itching. Cosmetics, articles of clothing, laundry products, family pets, pollens, or other allergens may be implicated. *Vernal conjunctivitis* presents in the spring and fall with itching (sometimes intense), foreign body sensation, tearing, light sensitivity, and ropy discharge. Occasionally it can cause damage to the cornea.

Contact lenses and their solutions can cause an infiltration of mast cells in the conjunctiva of the upper lid called *giant papillary conjunctivitis.* Discontinuing the lens usually resolves the problem promptly. If the skin around the affected eye is also red and swollen, the child may be having an allergic reaction to a topical medication.

The most serious form of allergic conjunctivitis is seen in *erythema multiforme,* or Stevens Johnson syndrome. The reaction in the conjunctiva to the inciting bacteria, virus or medication is similar to that seen in the skin and internal organs. Chronic scarring of the conjunctiva can destroy the cornea.

Treatment: Several treatments are available. Best, of course, is to remove the inciting cause. In many children, observation is sufficient. To some extent, all eyedrops are difficult, and the symptoms may simply not be bad enough to warrant the struggle. In other cases symptomatic relief can be obtained with ocular decongestants, such as naphazoline, tetrahydrozoline, or phenylephrine. These can be given as often as 4 times a day. Cromolyn and lodoxamide are mast-cell stabilizers that can be effective in some cases of vernal conjunctivitis, but they often must be given 4 to 6 times daily for several weeks before they work.

Two topical antihistamines have been every effective in the treatment of allergic conjunctivitis. Levocabastine (Livostin) is used four times a day and olopatadine (Patanol) is used twice a day. The medications are both well tolerated. They are continued for two weeks, then taken as needed. Ketorolac (Acular) is a nonsteroidal anti-inflammatory that can be used four times a day for a week or so. Only in unusually severe cases is it necessary to resort to topical steroids. Treatment of Stevens Johnson syndrome is merely supportive. Adhesions between the palpebral and bulbar conjunctiva (called *symblepharons*) may be broken with a glass rod or other surface.

When conjunctivitis becomes dangerous

Visual loss from conjunctivitis occurs most commonly when topical steroids are used improperly. These medications, often combined with antibiotics in eyedrops or ointments, can cause the spread of otherwise minor infections (especially corneal herpes), the formation of cataracts, and the development of glaucoma. They probably should only be administered by an ophthalmologist, who can monitor the eyes for complications.

Anyone wearing contact lenses who has redness or discomfort in the eyes should remove the lens promptly and consult an eye doctor if the symptoms don't clear within the first several hours.

The intact corneal barrier protects the eye from serious damage. But this barrier may be compromised by a corneal abrasion or scratch or by an overworn contact lens, for example. Then the risk of a corneal ulcer is much greater. Anyone wearing contact lenses who has redness or discomfort in the eyes should remove the lens promptly and consult an eye doctor if the symptoms don't clear within the first several hours. Until the corneal epithelium has recovered, the eye should be examined every day or two. Usually the healing is complete in a few days.

A form of chlamydial infection called *trachoma* is a serious problem. It is, in fact, one of the most common causes of blindness in the world, especially in Africa, the Middle East, India, and southeast Asia. The disease, which causes scarring of the conjunctiva and secondary damage to the cornea, is hardly ever seen in areas with adequate sanitation.

Is all pink eye conjunctivitis?

Conjunctivitis—viral, bacterial, or allergic—is by no means the only reason for eyes to become pink or inflamed. Other causes include iritis, infection or damage to the cornea, and inflammation of the tissues surrounding the eye.

Inflammation inside the eye, called *iritis* or *uveitis*, may be caused by a variety of systemic illnesses but is usually ideopathic. Usually the child complains of blurred vision, pain, or sensitivity to light. In chronic cases, though, the inflammation may smolder, causing damage inside of the eye with minimal symptoms, if any.

In cases of iritis, the conjunctival vessels may actually be normal, but deeper vessels in the episclera or the sclera are engorged. Eye doctors can tell the difference by looking with the slit lamp, which greatly magnifies the eye and may show inflammatory cells and protein (referred to as "cells and flare") in the anterior chamber or the vitreous.

Children with juvenile rheumatoid arthritis sometimes have iritis. They should be examined by an ophthalmologist periodically on a routine basis and should be seen urgently if the eyes are pink or if there are other visual symptoms.

A *corneal ulcer* is an infectious excavation of the cornea that usually looks like a small white spot. Ulcers can result from bacterial, viral or fungal infections. Intensive antimicrobial therapy is usually effective in stopping the infection, but scarring of the cornea may result in visual loss.

The differential diagnosis of pink eye includes poor eyelid closure, which exposes the cornea to drying, and inward misdirection of the lashes (called *trichiasis*), which can scratch the cornea. Lubricating drops or ointments can soothe and protect that sensitive structure, so eyelid surgery is only rarely needed.

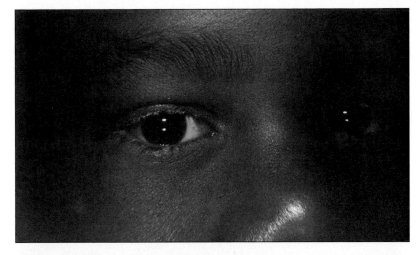

BLEPHARITIS. Often the result of staph infection, blepharitis causes mucopurulent debris to accumulate along the lashes.

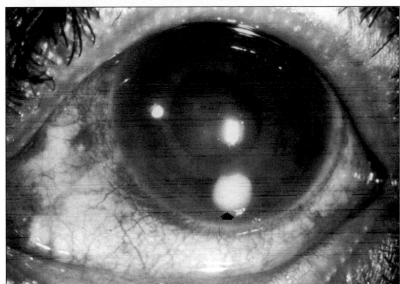

CORNEAL ULCER. Note the white spot in the cornea at the 5:30 position (arrow). The smaller white spots over the central pupil and at 9:00 are reflections from the camera flash.

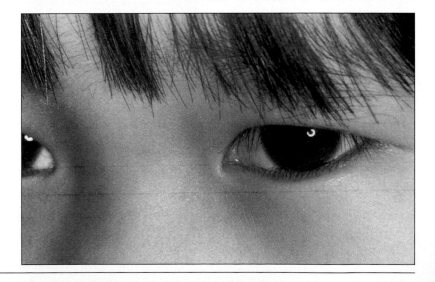

TRICHIASIS. The lashes are turned inward against the cornea. As a result, they can irritate the eye and cause tearing. (Photo courtesy Dale Meyer, MD)

STYE. More properly called a hordeolum, it is a small lid abscess. In this case there are two: one in the upper lid and a smaller one in the lower, both at the margins (arrows).

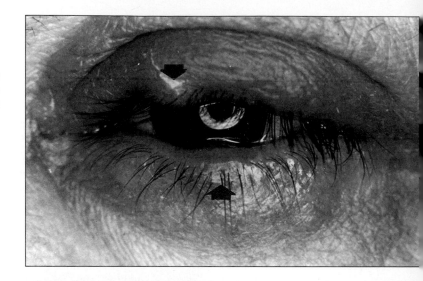

CHALAZION. Histopathologically a chalazion is a lipogranuloma. Unlike a stye, it is not red or painful.

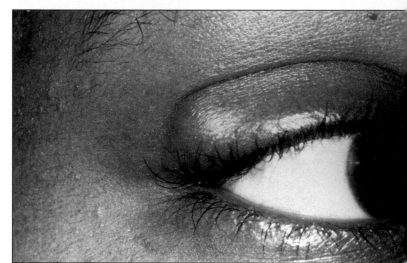

PERIORBITAL (PRESEPTAL) CELLULITIS. Note the diffuse swelling and redness of the lids. Involvement of the orbit itself can cause loss of ocular rotations, fever, and leukocytosis, and can have more serious sequellae. (Photo courtesy Jane Kivlin, MD)

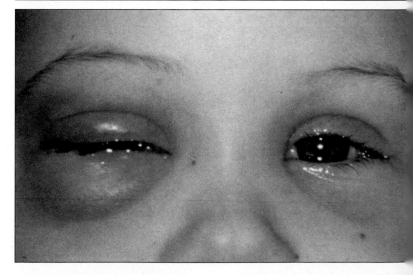

Inflammation of the eyelid (blepharitis) may take several forms, some of which are infectious. Seborrhea and staph infection are the most common causes of marginal blepharitis, centered along the lashes.

A *stye* is an infection of a tear gland in the eyelid, which causes localized pain, redness, swelling, and tenderness in the lid. Topical and oral antibiotics are usually curative. A more chronic inflammation of the same tear glands is called a *chalazion*, typically presenting as a non-tender lump in the lid. Both styes and chalazions are helped by warm compresses. Sometimes a chalazion takes weeks or even a few months to disappear, and may recur in another location. Occasionally it must be injected with steroids or surgically removed.

More diffuse inflammation of the eyelids is called *periorbital (preseptal) cellulitis*. It can be serious if it spreads into the orbit, behind the eye, because this area is so close to the brain. Often there is a history of trauma, an insect bite, or associated sinus infection. Preseptal cellulitis is sometimes treated with oral antibiotics, but orbital infections require hospitalization for intravenous therapy. The possibility of orbital abscess and rhabdomyosarcoma must be kept in mind.

Fortunately, Rebecca's story ends happily, as most do. By the next day, her eye was already beginning to get better, though her stuffy nose and sore throat kept her home for another day. She managed to avoid taking eyedrops altogether.

14 Blocked Tear Ducts: The Tearing (and Messy) Eye

In very young babies, blocked tear ducts are so common they can almost be considered normal.

Ben was fourteen months old when his mother took him to the ophthalmologist. Since birth, he had had a gooey yellow-green discharge from his left eye. At first it had come from both eyes, but then the right eye finally cleared when he was six months old. Ben's pediatrician had said he had a blocked tear duct and had prescribed an antibiotic eyedrop. But that hadn't seemed to help. So his parents learned to carry a box of tissues around to mop out his eye every hour or two. The eye also tended to look wet, as if it were always crying. His eyelids were often red and swollen.

Tears are necessary to keep the corneas comfortable, healthy and clear. They are made by glands located under the outer portions of the upper eyelids and along the inner surfaces of both the upper and lower lids. Then they are emptied onto the surface of the eyes, where they spread as a film over the corneas. This tear film is replenished with each blink.

Once they've done their job, the tears drain out of the eyes through a system of ducts that end up in the nose. That's why people have to blow their noses when they cry. These tear ducts are referred to as the lacrimal drainage system. The openings, at the upper end, are called *puncta* (singular, *punctum*), which are located at the eyelid margins near the inner corners of the upper and lower lids. After tears enter the puncta, they pass through the upper and lower *canaliculus* (plural *canaliculi*), literally "little canal," which runs more or less horizontally through the eyelid before emptying into the tear sac, or lacrimal sac, a little reservoir on the side of the nasal bridge. Next they go through the nasolacrimal duct, which passes through the bones beside the nose, and finally drain into in the nasal cavity.

A blockage anywhere in this drainage system will cause the tears to well up in the eyes, much as a blocked drain in the kitchen will cause water to back up in the sink.

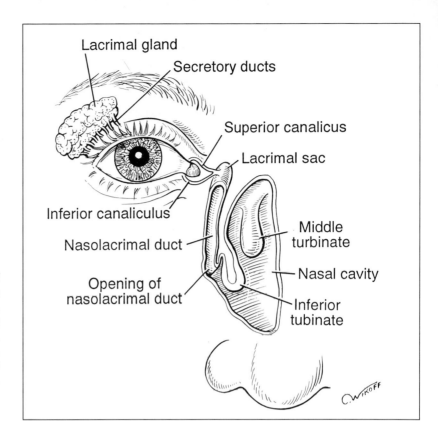

Lacrimal gland
Secretory ducts
Superior canalicus
Lacrimal sac
Inferior canaliculus
Middle turbinate
Nasolacrimal duct
Nasal cavity
Opening of nasolacrimal duct
Inferior tubinate

NASOLACRIMAL DRAINAGE SYSTEM (TEAR DUCT). Tears are formed in the lacrimal glands and wash over the eye. The lower lid acts like a rain gutter, directing the tears into the tiny canaliculi. After coursing into the lacrimal sac, they drain downward through the bony nasolacrimal duct into the nasal cavity.

What happens when tear drainage is blocked

Very often the tear ducts have not opened completely by the time a baby is born. Ben's problem is so common that it can almost be considered normal in very young babies. The blockage typically is caused by a thin membrane located near the bottom of the nasolacrimal duct, near the area where it empties into the nose. But it could be anywhere along the length of the tear ducts and cause the same symptoms Ben had.

When the tears can't get into the nose, they tend to spill onto the cheek and irritate the skin. It might be annoying for an infant to look through a "veil of tears," but blocked tear ducts don't seem to interfere with visual development.

Tears normally contain mucus. If the watery component of the tears evaporates, the mucus remains on the lashes and causes the lids to stick together in the morning. Specks of dried mucus may be seen around the lids and upper face. Because the lining of the lacrimal sac and the nasolacrimal duct is the same as the lining of the nose, it tends to swell and make more mucus when the baby has a cold. Swelling of the mucous membrane inside the nose may block the opening at the bottom of the duct. As a result, the discharge may be much worse until the infection clears.

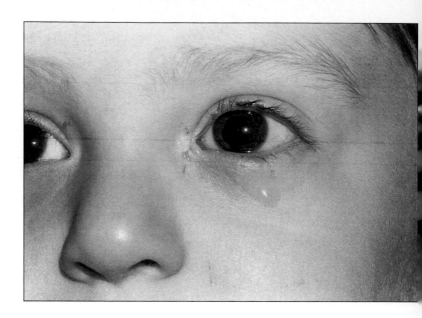

BLOCKED TEAR DUCT. This child's appearance is typical. The excess mucus may be more prominent than the excess tears.

Tear duct problems rarely, if ever, cause infection or other damage to the eyes. On the other hand, the blocked tears and mucus often become infected, and the infection certainly can "spill over" to involve the eyelids. Usually such an infection is not serious; it just causes a little redness and swelling around the lids. But occasionally it causes *cellulitis,* with the lids becoming very red and swollen shut. Infection in the lacrimal sac, called *dacryocystitis,* has similar symptoms, but the inflammation is localized to the area adjacent to the nasal bridge.

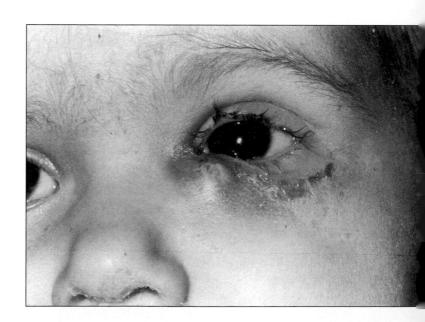

DACRYOCYSTITIS. There is an abscess involving the lacrimal sac, seen here as an inflamed mass in the inner portion of the lower lid.

MUCOCELE OF THE LACRIMAL SAC. This is an out-pouching of the sac, which is filled with mucus. There is typically an associated blockage of the tear duct. Secondary infection is common, presenting as a preseptal cellulitis.

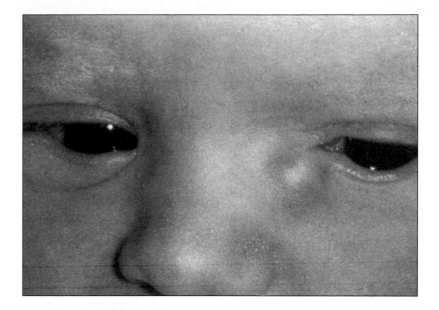

Infants who have a *mucocele*, a swelling of the lacrimal sac filled mostly with mucus, are particularly apt to have a problem with infections. A mucocele is usually noted at birth, but it may appear a week or so later as a round, bluish lump near the bridge of the nose. All children with mucoceles have blocked tear ducts, but only a few children with blocked tear ducts have mucoceles. Some children may even have an intranasal mucocele, which can cause trouble with breathing. Mucoceles may disappear on their own, but often they must be treated surgically.

Treatment for a blocked tear duct

The appropriate treatment for a blocked tear duct in one or both eyes depends on the age of the infant and on the severity of the symptoms. Since many blockages get better during the first months of life, most ophthalmologists tend to delay surgical treatment at first.

Massage   Eye doctors often recommend that the parents "massage" the infant's lacrimal sacs. This technique is simple: they press gently with a fingertip between the nasal bridge and the eye. Massage is repeated for several seconds 2 or more times a day. This may force blocked material out of the puncta and it can be wiped away. It is possible that the pressure will actually break open the membrane that is causing the blockage. Massage is especially helpful over a mucocele, which can accumulate immense amounts of mucus and tears.

Antibiotics   Antibiotic eyedrops and ointments seem to help control infections and reduce the amount of mucus. However, they do not cure the blockage itself. Most ophthalmologists recommend using the medication intermittently several times a day, but only when the lids are red and swollen or the discharge is particularly heavy. With overuse, some of these medications can themselves cause irritation.

Occasionally, antibiotic treatment may be given orally or even intravenously if swelling and redness of the lids indicate cellulitis or dacryocystitis. Systemic treatment should make the infection quickly resolve.

Lacrimal probing   Referral to an ophthalmologist is generally made when the symptoms are sufficient to warrant surgical treatment. Probing is usually easy and effective. In very young infants it may be performed without anesthesia in the doctor's office, but after the first few months it must be performed under anesthesia in an operating room.

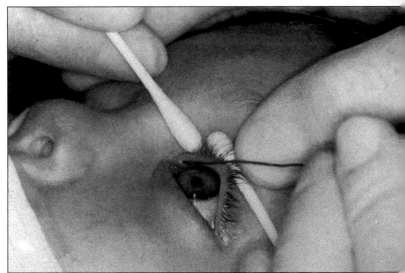

NASOLACRIMAL DUCT PROBING. The probe is introduced through the upper punctum, advanced through the upper canaliculus, and passed into the lacrimal sac. It is then directed downward, through the nasolacrimal duct and into the nose.

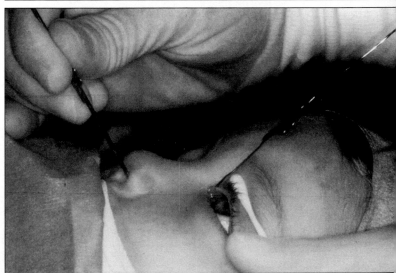

CONFIRMATION OF A SUCCESSFUL PROBING. A probe introduced through the nostril and beneath the inferior turbinate touches and moves the probe in the nasolacrimal duct.

A narrow wire called a *lacrimal probe* is pushed into the punctum and then down through the tear duct to break through the obstructing membrane. The probe is blunt and, because it goes through the punctum rather than through the skin, no cutting is required.

After the probing, some colored liquid may be squirted into the punctum and sucked out through the nose to be sure the system is open. Or a second probe, introduced through the nostril, may be used to touch the tip of the first probe before it's removed. The whole procedure takes only a few minutes, and complications are very rare. Typically a child wakes up from the anesthesia and is ready to leave the hospital within an hour after the procedure has been completed.

When should probing be done? Ophthalmologists do not agree as to the best time. Some doctors prefer to probe within a child's first few months of life because at this age the procedure can often take place in the doctor's office without general anesthesia. However, more than 90% of these children will get better without surgery by their first birthday. Therefore, many ophthalmologists prefer to wait until then.

The only disadvantage of waiting is that general anesthesia is required, increasing the expense and also the risk of surgery. We're both "late probers," feeling that children should be probed after they're a year old unless there is a problem due to a mucocele, a recurrent infection, or an unusually heavy discharge. But we can understand both points of view.

Outcome: Sometimes the procedure doesn't work. About 1 out of every 10 probings fails for reasons that are unknown. Some ophthalmologists believe they fail more often in children who are probed much later than age 1. Others fail because there is a problem in the nose. Perhaps the tissues lining the nose are swollen or the turbinate is too close to the lower opening of the tear duct. In these cases, surgically moving the cartilage aside can help. In other cases, repeating the probing later can work.

In some bilateral cases, one eye may clear completely after probing and yet the other may look just as gooey after surgery as before. Some eyes seem to improve after probing but are still not quite normal, and a slight discharge persists, especially when the child gets a cold. Sometimes it seems to take a week or two before the effect of the surgery can be seen. Usually, though, if the probing works, the discharge will not return.

Silicone intubation: If two or three probings (perhaps using a balloon catheter) and manipulations of the nasal cartilage fail, most ophthalmologists would recommend inserting a thin silicone tube to keep the tear duct open. The soft tube may be tied in place in the nose and it remains in the tear duct as long as several months. After it's removed, the tear duct will generally remain open.

Creating an opening: If even the tube fails, the next step is to perform an operation that requires cutting. Called a *dacryocysto-rhinostomy* (DCR), this procedure creates an internal opening between the lacrimal sac and the nose. Fortunately, children rarely need this type of surgery.

A blocked tear duct may require more than one operation to be cured. But it is truly exceptional for a person of any age to have to live with this kind of problem because it can't be repaired.

Other causes of tearing and messy eyes

Sometimes, a child will have discharge and tearing for reasons other than a blocked tear duct. In fact, anything that irritates the eye can be responsible:

• Misdirected eyelashes *(trichiasis)* rubbing against the cornea.

• Corneal abrasion, a foreign body in the eye, or any of a number of unusual corneal diseases.

• Inflammations of the conjunctiva or of the inside of the eye.

• Glaucoma (the most serious problem that masquerades as an obstructed tear duct).

Fortunately, all these problems have specific characteristics that help in distinguishing them from a blocked tear duct. Many cause the eye to become red and sensitive to light (not symptoms of a blocked tear duct). And because the reflex tears flow unimpeded into the nose, the child's nose may be always running. Children with blocked tear ducts tend to have dry noses, and their eyes are not light sensitive or inflamed.

Lack of tears

Some people are troubled because they have too few tears rather than too many. Their eyes may turn red, itch and burn, and may actually feel dry. In adults, especially women after menopause, it is due to inadequate tear formation. Some doctors treat such patients by intentionally blocking the tear ducts at the puncta. This problem is actually quite rare in children, although some children may not tear when they cry. Yet the eyes of these children suffer no ill effects.

15 Nystagmus: Eyes That Jiggle

It was hard for Jimmy's parents to describe, but his eyes were obviously not right. He just didn't seem to look at things the way other four-month-old babies do. His eyes were always roving back and forth. As the months passed, Jimmy's eyes didn't rove as far from side to side, but they continued to "jiggle" or "dance." Sometimes the movements were worse and other times they were better, but they never went away. Occasionally, Jimmy tended to nod his head rhythmically back and forth. And whenever he was concentrating on something—TV, for example—he would turn his face far to the right.

❧

Jimmy has *nystagmus* (nis-tag'-mus), an involuntary, repetitive movement of the eyes—usually both eyes— that usually begins during the first few months of life and is not likely ever to go away. In most cases the eyes move from side to side, though the movements can be vertical or circular. Their amplitude may become smaller during the first year.

Jimmy's parents reported that his eye movements seem to change from one moment to the next. Typically they get more noticeable when he is upset or tense or looking at a bright background, and they get better when he concentrates on something up close. They go away completely during sleep. These variations in movement are typical but the reasons for them are not well understood.

Nonvisual symptoms may be troublesome to children, especially during their teenage years when they are more conscious of their appearance. Parents will need to be supportive. If the nystagmus is severe, the child may appear to be scanning the visual environment. Some children are embarrassed by their eye movements or by their visual handicap and may therefore avoid eye contact with others. A prominent face turn may be cute in a young child, but it is not attractive in a young adult who has trouble facing the person he is talking to. A few children can feel the movement of their eyes, and that increases their self-consciousness.

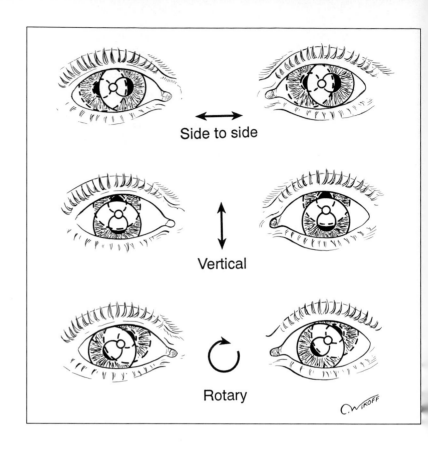

NYSTAGMUS. Nystagmus is repetitive involuntary movement of both eyes. Usually the movement is horizontal, but it may also be vertical or rotary.

Nystagmus and vision

For children with nystagmus, looking at something is like taking pictures very rapidly (several each second) with a camera that is shaking. Whenever the eye is still, when it is changing directions at the end of each movement, the brain can process a visual image. Amazing as it may seem, vision is blurred but it's not "jumpy" because the brain suppresses vision during the time the eyes move. (Adults with acquired nystagmus, as from neurologic conditions, are not so lucky. They complain of seeing movement in the environment, a symptom called *oscillopsia*.)

Children with nystagmus do not see normally, and the severity of the vision deficit depends in large part on how much the eyes move. Some children have less intense eye movements when they look far to one side. Jimmy found that he could see better by holding his face to the right (so his eyes were far to the left). Similarly, rhythmically nodding the head may partly compensate for the eye movements and permit better vision. These behaviors, which affect fewer than half of all children with nystagmus, are especially apt to occur when they are very interested in something that's hard to see. It's important that parents and teachers do not try to stop them from turning their face

Over time, the nystagmus and vision may both improve slightly, though nobody knows why.

or nodding their head, since either or both may help them see better. Children with mild nystagmus have only sight impairment of vision.

Almost always, nyatagmus interferes less with reading vision than distance vision. This is important for educational programming, since children with nystagmus usually learn to read well. Even with severe nystagmus and only 20/200 vision (or poorer), they can be excellent students. The services of a teacher of the visually impaired can be helpful, provided as a benefit to children who are declared "legally blind." Over time, the nystagmus and vision may both improve slightly, though nobody knows why.

As visual demands increase, an older student may find magnifying devices helpful for seeing the blackboard at school or for reading small print. The driver's test becomes an important concern for teenagers. Although they may not be able to read the 20/40 letters on the eye chart as most states require for an unrestricted license, they often will qualify for at least daytime driving.

Causes of nystagmus

Nystagmus is not usually hereditary; it typically happens to only one person in a family. In cases with underlying eye disorders, both dominant and recessive forms of hereditary transmission can occur. In most cases a cause is never found and the eyes are normal in all other respects. The most common diagnosis, therefore, is "idiopathic congenital nystagmus." Although the parents, the primary care physician, and the eye doctor may all feel better if there is a specific cause, it is actually better for the child if none is found. Children with idiopathic congenital nystagmus nearly always see fairly well.

Nystagmus probably results from a problem in the eye movement control system in the brainstem. The defect is usually not seen on CAT and MRI scans, nor is it detectable on postmortem examination. So it must be a functional abnormality at the cellular level.

Eye disorders Many disorders of the eyes can cause nystagmus, and so a major focus of the eye examination is to make certain that none of these is present. For example, children with congenital blindness due to severe disease anywhere in the eye may develop nystagmus during the first few months of life. Unfortunately, some of them are difficult to detect in early infancy.

Some examples of these problems include Leber's congenital amaurosis and other hereditary retinal diseases, retinopathy of prematurity, retinoblastoma, retinal and optic nerve colobomas, tumors and developmental defects of the optic nerve, and congenital cloudiness of the cornea.

Achromatopsia is an especially difficult diagnosis. This unusual disorder involving the color-sensitive photoreceptors (cones) in the retina may look exactly like idiopathic congenital nystagmus. When children are old enough to have color vision tested (age 4 to 6 or so), the diagnosis can be made easily because they will be found to have no color vision. Another characteristic of this condition is unusual sensitivity to light (photophobia).

Children with achromatopsia have a paradoxical pupillary response to dimming of the room lights. When the lights first go off, their pupils initally constrict rather than dilate. The mechanism of this "paradoxical pupil" is not clear. A type of special testing called *electro-retinography* is required to confirm the diagnosis. In this procedure, the electrical impulses generated in the retina when it is stimulated by light are measured with a contact-lens electrode. Because this test can be uncomfortable and inconclusive and because the condition has no treatment anyway, some ophthalmologists may prefer not to perform it unless a hereditary disorder is strongly suspected.

Systemic disorders   *Albinism* is probably the most common systemic disorder affecting the eyes that causes nystagmus. Almost everyone with albinism has nystagmus, probably because of an abnormality in the fovea, the central part of the retina. In severe cases the diagnosis is obvious from the white hair and pale skin. Light reflected from the back of the eyes may shine through the abnormally pigmented iris, and as a result the eyes may appear pink. Milder cases may not be apparent; a careful eye examination, including transillumination of the irides at the slit lamp, may be necessary for diagnosis.

Actually, albinism is a rather complicated condition involving more than the metabolism of melanin pigment in the eye, the skin, and the hair. Even in cases with apparent involvement of only the eyes, there is a higher-than-normal proportion of nerve fibers that cross the midline in the optic chiasm and in the auditory system. Rarely, albinos have other medical problems, such as a platelet function disorder that causes abnormal bleeding (Hermansky Pudlak syndrome) or a white blood cell disorder (Chediak Higashi syndrome) that predisposes to infections and tumors. By far the most important health problem albinos typically encounter is sun damage to their very sensitive skin. Social problems are more common among albinos whose families have skin that is darkly pigmented.

Brain disorders   In a small minority of cases, nystagmus may be caused by an identifiable problem in the brain. Children with cerebral palsy or other brain abnormalities have a higher incidence than other children. If a child develops nystagmus after the age of 6 months or so, the possibility of a brain tumor or other neurologic problem becomes a concern. Similarly, brain abnormalities should be considered if the nystagmus is unusual in any way: if it is episodic, if only one eye is affected, or if the eyes move in opposite directions. In such cases, or if there are symptoms such as headaches, seizures, personality changes, or the loss of developmental milestones, a neurologist should be consulted.

Special types of nystagmus

Spasmus nutans: this is a type of nystagmus involving very small and rapid eye movements. It begins when the infant is 6 to 12 months or so. Nodding and tilting of the head, with one ear toward the shoulder, are especially prominent in some of these children. Unlike idiopathic congenital nystagmus, which involves both eyes equally, spasmus nutans may be unilateral or asymmetric, involving just one eye or one eye much more than the other. Also unlike congenital nystagmus, it may completely disappear after a year or two.

In the past, ophthalmologists have tended to consider this a harmless condition and have not looked for underlying conditions. During the last several years, however, some children thought to have spasmus nutans have been found to have brain tumors. It is now recommended that children with this condition have CT or MRI scans and periodic eye examinations concentrating on the optic nerves and visual fields.

Latent nystagmus: In children with this fascinating condition, the eye movements are controlled, in some cases completely, until one eye is covered. Then nystagmus starts in both eyes. As long as both eyes are open, the vision is normal (or nearly normal, if there is still some nystagmus). But if you try to measure the vision in one eye at a time, the child will be unable to see nearly as well with either eye. Because their vision depends on having two eyes, children with this condition should always wear safety glasses for protection. Latent nystagmus is thought to occur only in children with idiopathic congenital nystagmus.

Treatment

Children with nystagmus are more likely to have strabismus, amblyopia, and refractive errors. These problems are all treatable in much the same way as in children without nystagmus.

It is important for parents to understand that glasses and patching will not normalize the vision, since these devices cannot take away the nystagmus itself. The idea is to improve vision to the best level possible, given the defect caused by the nystagmus.

For a child with accommodative esotropia, glasses may also help to align the eyes and may make the movements of the eyes less apparent to others. Adding a tint to the lenses may help. Eye muscle surgery can sometimes be very helpful: to correct strabismus, to improve abnormal head posture, and to lessen the nystagmus. Surgery is planned and executed just as for a child without nystagmus. (Interestingly, the eye movements stop while the child is under anesthesia.)

There is some evidence that esotropia is more common in children with nystagmus because the convergence of the eyes tends to dampen the eye movements. For children with this "nystagmus blockage syndrome," surgery for the strabismus does not make the nystagmus worse.

Head posture can be dramatically improved by eye muscle surgery. But it's important not to rush the surgery. Children should be consistently holding their head to the same side, the head posture should be easily apparent to the family, and it should be unimproved over several years. Severe head posturing is a serious handicap. Children may be unable to wear glasses, as the frames are designed for people who look straight ahead through the lenses rather than to the side. Deformities of the bones and joints in the neck may even develop from constantly turning to one side. Surgery can move the eyes so that the abnormal head posture is no longer apparent. An operation may also improve the nystagmus and the vision, but only slightly.

Surgery for children with normal head postures has been attempted. The theory is that a balanced weakening all of the horizontal rectus muscles may cause the eye movements to become less intense. The results of studies investigating this surgery are variable, and we do not recommend it at this time.

Because the eye movements seem to get worse in times of emotional stress, some have suggested using biofeedback to treat nystagmus. Others have considered ways to paralyze the eye muscles. In the future, these ideas may give rise to new treatments.

16 Cataracts

Mrs. Quinn was shocked when she was told that her three-month-old baby, Lisa, had cataracts. Mrs. Quinn's grandfather had undergone surgery for cataracts in his early 70s. Several of her grandparents' friends had had cataracts and all had been at least 60. So she had assumed that cataracts were part of growing older. Lisa was a healthy baby, slightly above the 70th percentile in both height and weight. But once the doctor told her about the cataracts, Mrs. Quinn remembered that her eye contact with Lisa during feeding had been less than with her other two children. When Lisa was about two months old, her eyes had started to jiggle, and this had led Mrs. Quinn and her husband to take their baby to an eye doctor. The doctor diagnosed the jiggling as nystagmus and also found the cataracts.

The lens is the transparent structure just behind the iris that focuses light onto the retina. It's normally hard to see because it is clear. If any part of the lens loses its transparency, becoming cloudy or opaque, that part is said to be a cataract. A cataract is not a growth *on* the lens; it's a loss of the clarity of the lens itself.

Cataracts are most common in older adults, but they can develop at any age. The symptoms vary depending on the stage of development, but the common denominator is poor vision. In Lisa's case the poor visual response was not noticed by her parents and caused no great concern until nystagmus started. Though nystagmus can occur with no apparent reason, it usually develops around 2 to 4 months of age in any infant who sees poorly from birth. It was the nystagmus that led to the discovery of Lisa's cataracts.

It is the combination of the location, the extent, and the degree of cloudiness that determines the effect of a cataract on the child's vision. The parents and the ophthalmologist usually share in evaluating the amount of visual impairment. The parents know how the child is functioning visually, and the ophthalmologist can examine the cataract itself. When a cataract is not be severe enough to interfere with vision significantly, surgery is not warranted. With time, however, it can become more dense or otherwise increase in severity, so periodic reevaluations will be needed.

What causes cataracts in children?

When Mrs. Quinn was told that Lisa had cataracts, she responded like every other parent. She wanted to know what had caused her child to get them. Had she done something wrong? Had she eaten the wrong food or lifted something too heavy while she was carrying her baby?

In an otherwise healthy infant or child who is growing and developing normally, the cause of the cataracts is almost never found. Most occur for no apparent reason. If we knew why they occur, perhaps a way could be found to prevent them.

In children who are otherwise apparently healthy, the most common single cause is probably heredity. Cataracts are usually passed from one generation to the next as an autosomal dominant trait. Often, there is variable expression in different family members: one parent may have a mild cataract in one eye from birth, yet pass on dense bilateral cataracts to the next generation. A careful history and examination of family members should make the diagnosis possible.

Many childhood conditions can be associated with cataracts. Nearly all have a severe effect on the health and well-being of the child. They are so severe and so apparent that the parents and the primary care physician easily recognize that something is wrong, and appropriate tests and consultations will permit diagnosis and direct appropriate treatment.

POSSIBLE CAUSES OF CATARACTS IN INFANTS AND CHILDREN
1. Heredity (usually autosomal dominant)
2. Intrauterine infection: TORCH organisms
3. Metabolic disorders: galactosemia, hypoparathyroidism, pseudo-hypoparathyroidism, diabetes mellitus, Lowe (oculo-cerebro-renal) syndrome, Alport (familial hemorrhagic nephritis) syndrome
4. Chromosomal disorders
5. Systemic syndromes: Hallermann-Streiff-Conradi, myotonicdystrophy, Stickler, Cockayne, Rubenstein-Taybi
6. Dermatologic disorders: ichthyosis, ectodermal dysplasia, incontinentia pigmenti
7. Craniofacial dysostoses
8. Prematurity

Adapted from *Pediatric Ophthalmology, 3nd ed.* by Nelson, Calhoun and Harley, © 1991 by W. B. Saunders. Co.

Another cause is congenital infection with the "TORCH" organisms (including toxoplasmosis, rubella, cytomegalovirus, and herpes simplex). Titers for these organisms can be helpful. There are usually other systemic manifestations of these conditions.

Metabolic disorders—galactosemia, for example—can present with bilateral cataracts as an isolated finding if the enzyme missing is galactokinase. The classic form, involving galactose-1-phosphate uridyl transferase, causes more obvious systemic involvement. Specific enzyme assays should help with this diagnosis. Disorders of calcium and phosphorus metabolism and childhood diabetes may also be associated with cataracts, but these are not the presenting sign.

Uveitis or iritis, inflammation inside the eye, can cause cataracts, especially in older children. Such inflammation can be practically asymptomatic, especially if associated with juvenile rheumatoid arthritis or sarcoidosis.

Finally, it is important not to forget trauma. Ocular penetration with sharp objects or small missiles can cause cataracts with little external evidence. Cases of child abuse may be particularly difficult to recognize. Other associations, not strictly causal, are rare.

How is a cataract detected in a child?

Most commonly, the parents see a white spot when they look at the pupil. A cataract is nearly always white or light gray, and this color may be apparent in the normally black pupil. The primary care physician may detect the opacity in the red pupillary reflex by looking through the ophthalmoscope. Or the cataract may be similarly apparent in photographs.

Unilateral cataract　In about half of all children with cataracts, only one eye is affected. Such babies seem to see normally because of the good vision in the other eye, and both eyes may follow normally. Neither the parents nor the pediatrician have any reason to think there is an eye problem. It may be difficult to evaluate the small pupils of infants, who tend to keep their eyes closed. But eventually the problem will be noticed by someone.

One common way that a cataract is discovered is from the development of strabismus in that eye. If one eye does not see well for any reason—for the purposes of this chapter, because of a cataract—it will often not stay aligned with the normal eye. It may turn in, turn out, or even turn up. The deviation may be easily seen by the family, and the subsequent eye examination will reveal the cataract.

In older children, vision screenings or measurements of the vision in each eye will identify poor vision in one eye compared to the other,

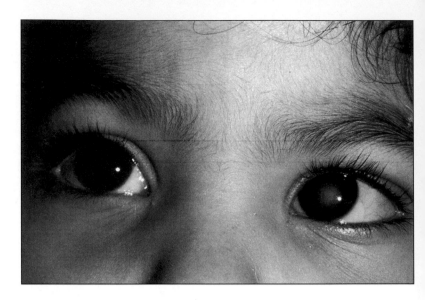

CATARACT AND ESOTROPIA. Note the gray discoloration in the left pupil. This child's cataract caused poor vision in the left eye, which then turned inward.

leading to an eye examination that reveals the cataract. Unfortunately, such screenings are often not performed until a child is kindergarten age.

Bilateral cataracts   In unrecognized cases, parents may begin to observe the behavioral effects of their child's poor vision. An infant with severe cataracts in both eyes may have trouble looking at a parent's face, smiling in response to a smile, or following a moving parent with the eyes. As in Lisa's case, nystagmus may develop. An older child may struggle to find familiar things, collide with obstacles, or hold objects very close.

Surgery

If the cataract has progressed sufficiently to interfere with vision, something must be done. Making the pupil larger with eyedrops so the child can "see around" the cataract(s) is occasionally helpful, but nearly all severe cases require surgery to remove the cataract.

Even though only a portion of the lens may be cloudy, while the rest of the lens is clear and otherwise normal, the entire lens must be removed. (There is no way to change the cloudy portion back to its normal clarity.) The ophthalmologist makes an incision in the eye that is several millimeters long, then uses a small instrument that liquifies the lens or cuts it into tiny pieces so that it can be vacuumed out of the eye. An intraocular lens may then be implanted *(see below).* To magnify the eye during surgery the ophthalmologist uses an operating microscope. The incision is closed with sutures that are finer than a human hair, so fine that the child can't feel them.

CATARACT SURGERY

To remove the cataract, the surgeon inserts a small instrument into the eye through an incision near the edge of the cornea.

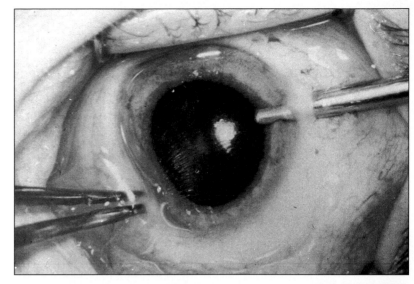

As the surgery progresses, tiny bits of the cataractous lens are vacuumed out of the eye. An intraocular lens may then be implanted in certain cases.

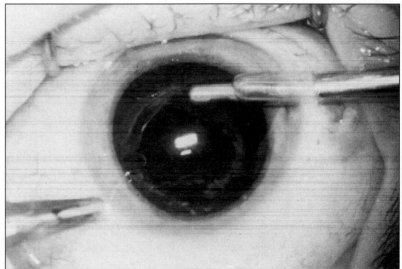

These days, most cataract surgery—in all but the youngest infants—is done on an outpatient basis. Very young or premature babies may require observation in the hospital overnight after having general anesthesia. But most children are brought to the hospital only for the day of their surgery, which takes about an hour. After the procedure the eye is covered with a patch.

Recovery from anesthesia takes several hours, after which the child can be taken home. Normal feedings are gradually restored, and there are only minimal restrictions on normal activities. Eyedrops may be prescribed to keep the pupil dilated and to minimize inflammation, and the parents are asked to bring the child back to the doctor's office for examinations at specified intervals for a month or so.

Restoring vision after surgery

Once the cataract has been removed, the eye can see only blurred images. The optical function of the lens must be replaced by an artificial lens in one of three places: in front of the eye in the form of glasses, on the eye in the form of a contact lens, or within the eye in the form of an intraocular lens. Each has its advantages and disadvantages, its advocates and detractors.

Glasses   To replace the entire optical function of the lens that is removed, glasses must be very strong, which also means thick and heavy. Many children opt for contact lenses when they become aware that they look different from their peers. But glasses may be preferable for others, particularly preschool children, who are too young to want contact lenses and too old and strong to allow their parents to put contacts in each morning and remove them each night.

Thinner, "regular-looking" glasses are frequently used to obtain the best possible vision for a child who has a contact lens or an intraocular lens that is not exactly the right power. (Sometimes the lenses are not available in exactly the correct power, or some astigmatism may remain even with the contacts in place.) The glasses may have bifocal lenses, ground to one strength in the upper portion for seeing at a distance and to a higher strength below for seeing close.

Contact lenses   Contact lenses rest on the front surface of the eye, the cornea. The lenses actually float on a thin layer of tears. There are three general types: hard, soft, and rigid gas-permeable. In the last decade or so, nearly all contact lenses have been of the latter two types. Soft contacts are usually better tolerated by the wearer, so a long adaptation process is not needed. Gas-permeable lenses are easier to care for and they correct astigmatism better.

Regardless of the specific type prescribed, the parents must be careful to clean and sterilize the lenses according to the instructions given by the doctor who fits them. Contact lenses can predispose the eyes to infections of the cornea, which can be mild, or so serious as to be potentially blinding.

When an infant has a cataract removed, the optical defect is usually corrected with "continuous-wear" soft contact lenses. The lenses are not really worn continuously, but remain in the eye for several days at a time between cleanings. When the child is older, these are generally replaced by daily-wear lenses, which are removed every night for sterilizing, then put back into the eyes the next day. The major reason for this switch to the extra burden of daily-wear lenses is that nightly sterilization reduces the chance of infection.

Intraocular lenses   An intraocular lens (IOL) is placed within the eye, usually just behind the iris in the same location that the natural lens occupied. This option is the nearly universal choice for adults who have cataracts removed, and it is gradually becoming more accepted for older children. The question among ophthalmologists has to do with exactly when a child is "older." That decision is based to a large extent on when the eyes stop growing.

The eye, like the brain, grows rapidly for the first several years after birth, so that by the time a child is 2 or 3 most of the growth has taken place. Growth changes occur thereafter, but at a much slower rate. Because the eye's prescription changes as it grows, an IOL should not be inserted until most of this growth is finished. An IOL cannot be changed easily, like glasses or contact lenses, and it is important that its power be appropriate for a lifetime.

The IOL is normally placed in the eye at the time of cataract removal. Its correct power is determined by measurements of the front curve of the cornea by keratometry and of the axial (front-to-back) length of the eye by ultrasonography. Both of these are painless

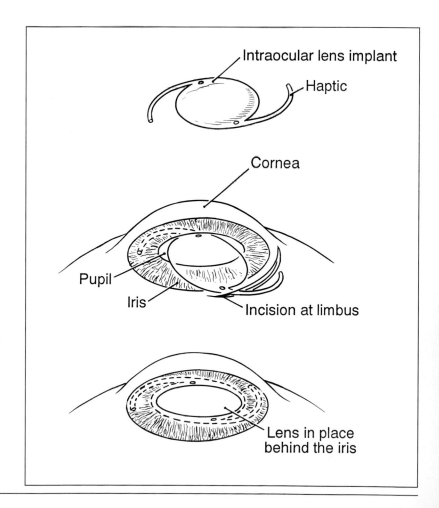

INTRAOCULAR LENS (IOL) IMPLANTATION. The top picture shows the plastic IOL. The middle picture shows the IOL being implanted behind the iris through the same small incision used to remove the cataract. The bottom picture shows how the haptics stabilize the lens, ideally within the lens capsule.

techniques performed in the doctor's office before surgery.

IOL surgery: The natural lens is surrounded by a transparent covering called the *capsule*. The anterior capsule is just behind the iris. The anterior and posterior capsule meet at the edge of the lens, sometimes called the *equator*.

During surgery the central portion of the anterior capsule is removed through the pupil, which has been dilated with eyedrops. The posterior capsule and the periphery of the anterior capsule may be left intact in order to create a bag into which the IOL is placed. The IOL has little plastic extensions called *haptics* that fit into the capsule and press against its equator to hold the optical portion of the IOL in place behind the pupil.

Even though the posterior capsule is clear at the time of surgery, it generally loses that clarity in a matter of months to years. This problem is especially common in children. As a result, the clear vision that was obtained several weeks after surgery is slowly reduced. In adults and in children who are old enough to sit still for several minutes, a laser can be used to make a small hole in the cloudy posterior capsule. In children who are too young to sit still for this procedure, a small hole is often made in the posterior capsule at the time of surgery. The posterior capsule around this hole may still become cloudy, but the hole is big enough to see through.

The outcome of surgery

Cataract surgery in children, as in adults, is remarkably effective. The surgery itself is almost always a success.

Problems that can develop Sometimes removing the cloudy lens is difficult, and the iris can be damaged. If the lens capsule is torn, it may be impossible to implant an IOL. There are even rare cases of retinal injury or devastating infection *(endophthalmitis)* that can rob the eye of vision. But such problems are exceptional.

Children who undergo cataract surgery rarely see normally, even with optical correction. The main obstacle is amblyopia. Especially when only one eye had a cataract, the other eye sees so well that the eye that had the cataract may remain "lazy." Part-time patching throughout early childhood can help make them use the operated eye. Amblyopia can also affect children who have surgery on both eyes, partly as a result of the blurred image caused by the cataracts. Patching helps such children only if one eye is more amblyopic than the other.

Over the months and years following surgery, other problems may emerge. Most children develop strabismus in the eye with poorer vision (it may either cross in or turn out). Eye muscle surgery is usually successful. Sometimes the cataract returns; it may be visible as a gray spot in the pupil. This complication usually shows up within 6 months after surgery and in some ways resembles scar tissue within the eye. It can usually be removed by additional surgery.

A more disturbing complication is the development of glaucoma, typically several years after apparently successful surgery. The high pressure inside the eye is usually not detectable except on careful examination, and it is difficult to measure the eye pressure of young children without general anesthesia. The ophthalmologist will therefore look for other indications, such as damage to the optic nerve, increase in the size of the cornea, and overly rapid decrease in the strength of the optical correction. Although glaucoma sometimes requires surgery, many children can be treated with eyedrops alone.

The visual outcome   The visual outcome depends on the severity of the amblyopia and any other complications that may develop. Vision is likely to be poor if the child cannot tolerate the recommended patching and optical correction, if there is a delay in removing a severe cataract, or if glaucoma sets in and is not treated. Children with late-onset cataracts do the best, since their eyes learn to see before the cataract begins to obscure their vision. Indeed, some see almost normally. The average child may see between 20/60 and 20/200—well enough to function well in school and in most activities. One of the most important factors in determining a favorable outcome is regular, routine follow-ups throughout childhood.

17 Glaucoma

There was definitely something wrong with Jared's eyes. When his parents first brought him home from the hospital, his eyes teared a lot, even when he wasn't crying. Later, when he was exposed to bright light, he would squeeze his eyes closed or hide them with his hands, and his eyes would tear even more. At first his parents thought he was just shy. But even the overhead light in his bedroom bothered him, and he would cry when he was outdoors on a sunny day. Everybody his parents talked to told them that tearing was normal for babies and that Jared would "grow out of it." But the problem kept getting worse. Then one day Jared's left eye became cloudy-looking. Alarmed, his parents took him to the pediatrician, who referred them to an ophthalmologist.

Jared has glaucoma, a disease that children rarely get. Glaucoma affects only about one infant in 10,000. When it does occur, it usually begins before birth or shortly after birth; except in children who have had cataract surgery, it is very unusual after the first year. Glaucoma can affect one or both eyes. Unlike adults, children with glaucoma almost always have symptoms, and Jared's are typical.

What is glaucoma?

Glaucoma is a disorder in which the pressure inside the eye is too high. Left untreated, it gradually and irreversibly damages the optic nerve and can result in blindness.

Most people think of glaucoma as a disease of older people, largely because the majority of cases develop after age 40 or 50. Even though medical and surgical treatment is usually effective, glaucoma is a particularly dangerous disease in adults because there are no symptoms. The pressure first damages only the peripheral parts of the field of vision and the effects of this damage can go unnoticed. As a result,

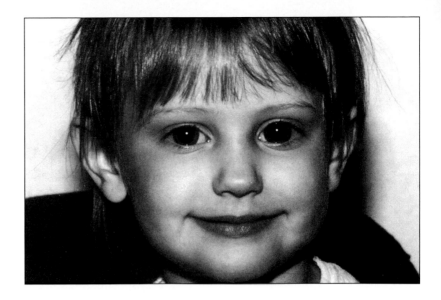

UNILATERAL GLAUCOMA, LEFT EYE. Note the larger corneal (or iris) diameter in the left eye. This eye is pushing the lids farther apart so that the left lid fissure is larger. A difference in size between the two eyes suggests there may be glaucoma in the larger eye, unless the other eye is abnormally small.

many don't find out that they have a problem until the disease is advanced. Fortunately, children with glaucoma are usually brought to medical attention because of light sensitivity, tearing, enlargement of the eye, or corneal couding.

In both children and adults, there is a defect in the way the aqueous humor drains out of the eye. The aqueous is the watery fluid that fills the front part of the eye. The exact nature of this defect is usually unknown. It is not related to blood pressure, as many people think. The pressure inside the eye increases because the ciliary body continues to make aqueous, which doesn't flow out of the eye as it normally should.

The effect of glaucoma on vision   As the disease progresses, aqueous may begin to leak into the cornea, causing it to become edematous and hazy. The child's vision is affected because looking through the haze is like looking through a translucent shower curtain.

If one eye is involved, that eye may develop strabismus. (Any time one eye does not see well for any reason, it may not stay aligned with the normal eye.) When both eyes are affected, the child may develop nystagmus, or may simply not see well.

Eyeball enlargement and related symptoms   The eyes of adults are rigid, so they stay the same size while the pressure inside them increases. But children's eyes are distensible, and when the pressure inside is too high they tend to enlarge, much like a balloon that is filled with water. The enlargement produces its most dramatic effects on the cornea, partly because that part of the eye is stretched the most. As it enlarges, minute cracks, called *Haab's striae*, develop in the inner layer of the cornea, *Descemet's membrane*.

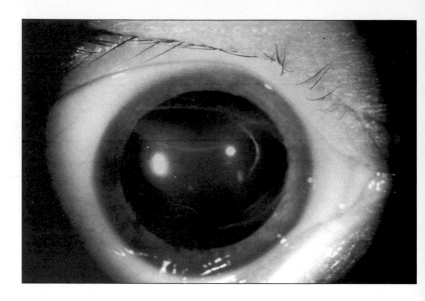

BREAKS IN DESCEMET'S MEMBRANE. The irregular gray lines running running roughly horizontally represent breaks in Descemet's membrane, one of the inner layers of the cornea. In this case, the breaks resulted from stretching or enlarging of the eye from glaucoma. Note the mild haze from corneal edema. (Photo courtesy Michael Belin MD)

As the high pressure forces aqueous to leak into the cornea, microscopic bubbles *(bullae)* are formed on the front surface. These bullae are thin-walled, so they are broken easily, just by blinking or moving the eyes. Once they are broken they act like multiple tiny scratches on the cornea, producing the symptoms of a foreign body, including photophobia. In some cases even normal room light can be uncomfortable, causing the eyes to tear and the child to squeeze the eyes tightly closed. Sunlight is downright painful.

The eye also stretches toward the back, away from the cornea. The symptoms of this backward stretching are not so obvious. But elongation of the eye results in myopia. Actually it is quite unusual for children with glaucoma not to be nearsighted, and typically their prescriptions are quite strong. In fact, one millimeter of elongation is equivalent to about 3 or 4 diopters of myopia, more than enough to blur a child's uncorrected vision to the level of legal blindness.

Over time, the enlargement of the eye may become more apparent. The cornea, about 10 mm in diameter at birth, normally grows to about 11.5 mm—nearly adult size—by the second birthday. Without treatment, glaucoma can enlarge the cornea to 17 mm or more. An old name for this condition is *buphthalmos*, which is the Greek word meaning "ox eye."

So, in addition to being blind and painful, eyes with severe glaucoma can be unsightly as well. Mild degrees of enlargement may at first escape detection, especially if both eyes are equally involved. The child's "beautiful big eyes" may even be an attractive feature. If one eye is larger than the other, the difference will be more easily recognized as an abnormality.

Other conditions associated with glaucoma

In most cases, glaucoma in childhood is an isolated problem. The few exceptions are associated with any of a long list of other conditions. Children known to have any of these should be examined for glaucoma carefully and at regular intervals.

Because many of these conditions are quite rare, only a few will be discussed here.

Systemic conditions affecting the eyes   *Sturge-Weber syndrome* is characterized by a red birthmark on the child's face, usually stopping abruptly at the midline. It may be accompanied by a seizure disorder, sometimes with developmental impairment and weakness of specific body parts. The birthmark, which is called a "port wine stain" *(nevus flammeus)*, is actually a collection of abnormal blood vessels. If these involve the upper eyelid, they may also extend beneath the conjunctiva, where they may interfere with the drainage of aqueous humor and cause a particularly difficult form of glaucoma.

Neurofibromatosis, or *von Recklinghausen's disease,* is an autosomal dominant disease of variable severity. Most cases are mild, and the affected child may have only a few light brown birthmarks ("cafe-au-lait spots") on the skin. A severely affected child may also have disfiguring tumors throughout the body and in the central nervous system, as well as other changes in and around the eyes. Although most children with this disease do not have glaucoma, they are significantly more at risk than other children.

Rieger and Lowe syndromes are both also hereditary. Rieger syndrome (autosomal dominant) includes abnormalities of the iris and irregular formation of the teeth and bones. The pupils may be mis-

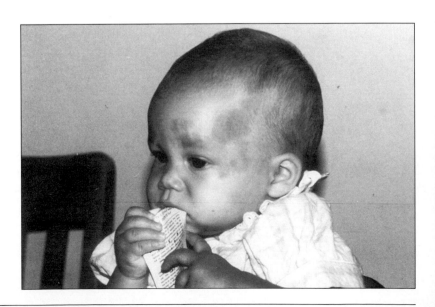

STURGE WEBER SYNDROME. The characteristic "port wine stain" birthmark may be associated with glaucoma on the same side.

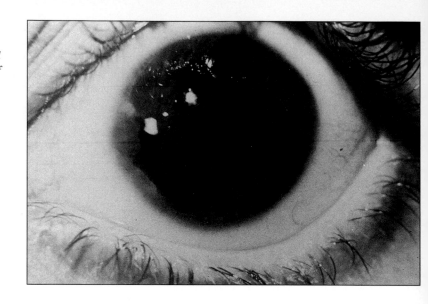

RIEGER SYNDROME. This congenital anomaly of the iris presents a risk of glaucoma.

shapen or misplaced. Lowe syndrome, which usually affects boys (x-linked recessive), includes childhood cataracts, developmental delay, and abnormal kidney function. Children with either syndrome may develop glaucoma in the first few years of life.

Conditions limited to the eyes   Children with *aniridia* have hardly any iris tissue; it may appear to be absent altogether. Parents may notice that the eyes are dark. However, what appears to be dark is actually a very widely "dilated" pupil. A child with aniridia may also have cloudy corneas, cataracts, nystagmus, and poor vision. Glaucoma may develop because the poorly formed iris tends to interfere with the drainage of aqueous humor. Aniridia may run in families (autosomal dominant), but is most often sporadic.

When there is no family history of aniridia, there is a substantial risk (about 1 in 5) of a *Wilm's tumor* in the kidney, but for unknown reasons there is no increased risk in those with a family history of the disease. Wilm's tumor is better treated in its early stages; therefore children with aniridia should be examined for this problem at regular intervals. No treatment is necessary for the aniridia itself. The other eye problems associated with it are often treatable, and patients can usually expect a lifetime of reasonable vision (20/200 or better).

Peter and Axenfeld syndromes are part of a group of disorders affecting the formation of the front part of the eye, and they are all associated with an increased risk of glaucoma. Each has slightly different features, but all may involve abnormalities of the angle between the iris and the cornea where aqueous humor is drained from the eye. A child with Peter syndrome, for example, has a cloudy spot in the cornea that may be connected to the iris by strands of pigmented tissue. In rare cases, the clouding may be severe enough to require

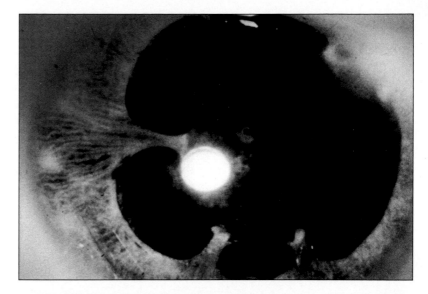

PETER SYNDROME. A localized opacity in the posterior cornea may be connected to the iris by strands of pigmented tissue. In rare cases, the opacity is severe enough to require corneal transplantation.

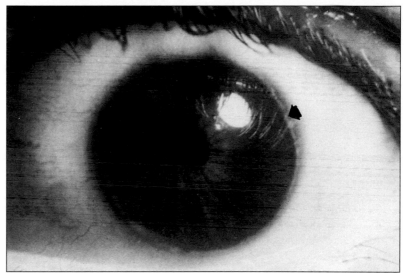

AXENFELD SYNDROME. The arrow indicates a gray ring just inside the limbus (the junction of the cornea and sclera). This ring, called Axenfeld anomaly, marks the edge of Descemet membrane. In Axenfeld syndrome, there are pigmented iris strands extending to this ring and an associated risk of glaucoma.

corneal transplantation. Axenfeld syndrome also involves pigmented attachments between the iris and the cornea, but they are far from the pupil, and the cornea remains clear. Both Peter and Axenfeld syndromes have some of the features of Rieger syndrome, which was mentioned above.

Examining the eye for glaucoma

In a cooperative adult, the intraocular pressure can be measured easily and painlessly with any of a variety of devices called *tonometers*. The angle between the iris and the cornea, where the fluid drains out of the eye, is examined using a special contact lens called a *gonioscope*. The optic nerve and the damage that has been done to it can

TONOMETRY. Sometimes infants will permit measurement of the pressure within the eye using a hand-held instrument called a tonometer. Often, sedation or general anesthesia is required.

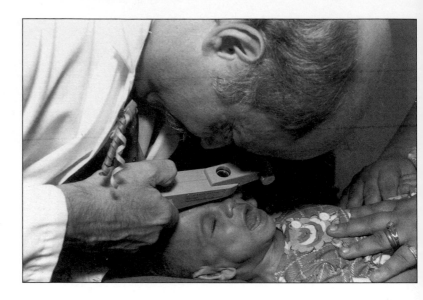

be seen by looking through the pupil with an *ophthalmoscope*, and then studied, photographed, and even analyzed with a computer. Damage to the peripheral vision can be measured with a *visual field test*.

It is simply impossible, however, to examine a young child in most of these ways. Even measuring the pressure of the eye, the most direct assessment of glaucoma, can be difficult. A small baby may be approached with a hand-held tonometer while taking a bottle. A less cooperative child up to age 4 or even older may require general anesthesia. Unfortunately, measuring the pressure under anesthesia often gives falsely low readings. But anesthesia does permit the careful measurement of the cornea's diameter, microscopic assessment for Haab's striae or associated abnormalities in the front part of the eye, examination of the drainage angle, and study of the optic nerve. Usually children are not sufficiently attentive to respond to a visual field test until they are well into elementary school.

As stated, glaucoma is a rare disease in children, and they are not specifically tested for it unless they display symptoms such as light sensitivity, asymmetry or enlarged corneas, etc. Such symptoms warrant referral to an ophthalmologist. Then, based on the parents' observations and on the office examination, the ophthalmologist will decide whether to examine the eyes under anesthesia, and will use these findings to decide whether surgery is needed. In some cases, children are followed for several weeks, or even several months, to check for any signs of progression before a decision is made.

Treatment

Glaucoma in adults is treated with medicines more often than is childhood glaucoma. Not only do the medications not seem to work as well in children, it is difficult for a child to use oral medications or eyedrops, typically two to four times a day, for an indefinite period of time.

Children may be given medical treatment, however, either before surgery, as a temporizing measure, or after surgery, to augment its effect. Some of the topical medications are adrenergic agonists (epinephrine, propine, apraclonidine, brimonidine), or antagonists (timolol, levobunolol, betaxolol). Others are cholinergics (carbachol, pilocarpine, physoltigmine, echothiophate). Latanoprost is a prostoglandin analog. All lower the intraocular pressure either by interfering with the production of aqueous humor or by speeding its drainage from the eye.

Hyperosmotic agents, given systemically, can lower the pressure rapidly, but generally for only a short time. These include oral glycerine and isosorbide and intravenous mannitol. One of the most effective systemic treatments, which can be given on a long-term basis, is acetazolamide. This carbonic anhydrase inhibitor decreases aqueous production, but it can cause a metabolic acidosis requiring sodium bicarbonate. Dorzolamide, a topical carbonic anhydrase inhibitor, is less likely to produce this side effect.

GONIOTOMY. This is often the first surgical procedure performed for children with glaucoma. In this example, the knife is used inside the eye to incise the angle between the iris and the cornea for 100 degrees. The surgeon looks into the angle using an instrument called a gonioscope.

Surgical treatment is designed to normalize the intraocular pressure permanently, preventing further damage to the optic nerve. In the most widely performed procedure, *goniotomy*, the surgeon makes an incision into the drainage angle. In some cases, especially if the cornea is so hazy that the angle can't be seen well, a *trabeculotomy* or *trabeculectomy* may be substituted. Both of these involve making an opening into the angle from outside the eye. All three of these surgical procedures are intended to improve the drainage of aqueous humor.

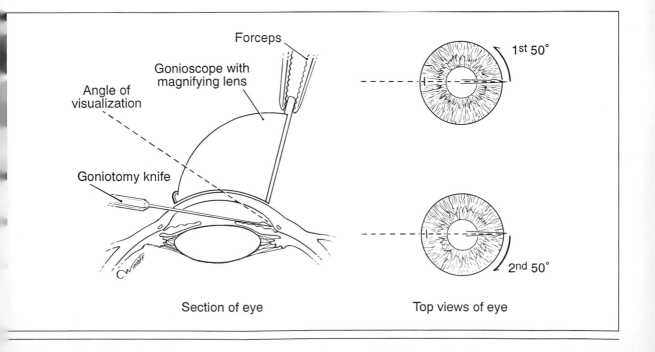

Forceps

Gonioscope with magnifying lens

Angle of visualization

Goniotomy knife

1st 50°

2nd 50°

Section of eye

Top views of eye

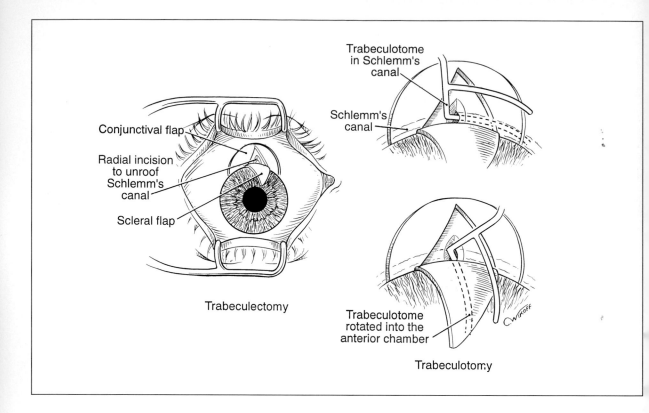

Conjunctival flap

Radial incision
to unroof
Schlemm's
canal

Scleral flap

Trabeculectomy

Trabeculotome
in Schlemm's
canal

Schlemm's
canal

Trabeculotome
rotated into the
anterior chamber

Trabeculotomy

TRABECULECTOMY AND TRABECULO-
TOMY. These are two surgical options
often used to improve drainage of aque-
ous when goniotomy is not feasible.
In a trabeculectomy (left), the surgeon
opens a partial thickness flap of sclera
which allows aqueous to drain under
the conjunctiva. In this case, a trabecu-
lotomy (right) is also being performed.
In this procedure, a trabeculotome is
passed into Schlemm's canal, then
rotated through the trabecular mesh-
work into the anterior chamber.

Laser treatments have been successful in accomplishing the same goal in adults, though they have not been used as often in children. If other surgical approaches fail, a portion of the ciliary body may be treated by freezing or laser in order to decrease the production of aqueous humor.

Outcome

Visual outcome may be limited by amblyopia, especially when the glaucoma is in one eye or unequally in both eyes. Such children require close monitoring of their glasses prescriptions and may need patching as well.

The prognosis depends on a number of factors. If the pressure cannot be brought under effective control, if the disease was present at birth, if it became severe before the diagnosis was made, or if it is associated with other malformations of the eye, the outlook for visual recovery may be poor. But even in severe cases the pressure can usually be controlled with one or more of the surgical procedures described above. And in some more favorable cases, with milder involvement and prompt, effective therapy, visual recovery may be nearly normal.

18 Some Structural Disorders of the Visual System

Ophthalmology textbooks describe literally hundreds of medical conditions that can cause visual deficits in children. It is impossible to cover them all in a book of this length. The most important have been addressed in previous chapters. But there are several more that are common enough to deserve mention.

Ptosis

Drooping of the upper eyelid is called *blepharoptosis*, or ptosis for short. It is a common congenital problem that can affect one or both eyes, for which there is usually no known cause. It can run in families. Weakness in other muscles can occur, but less commonly in children than in adults. In some children the position of the lid is affected by movements of the mouth, as in feeding; this association is called *Marcus Gunn jaw-winking*. In other children the eyelid only looks lower because the eye itself is lower. Many other abnormalities of eyelid position and shape occur less commonly.

Eyelid surgery, the only remedy, can be performed at any age.

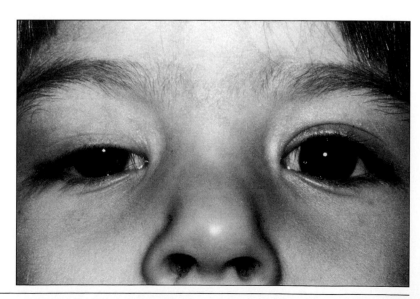

PTOSIS. In this case of congenital ptosis, only the right eye was affected. Surgery is usually delayed until age 2 to 4 years, unless the lids are so badly closed as to threaten visual loss from amblyopia. (Photo courtesy Dale Meyer, MD)

153

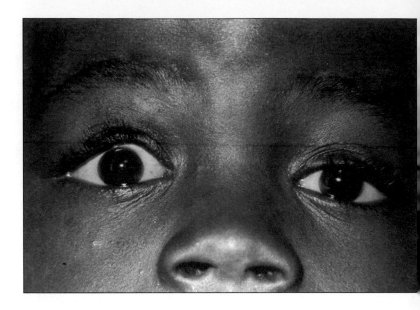

PTOSIS OVERCORRECTION. The right upper lid has been raised too much by surgery to correct ptosis.

Ptosis may improve slightly as the face grows, so surgery is usually delayed at least until a child is 2 to 4 years of age unless the problem is unusually severe. For example, a child may be forced to raise the chin in order to look out from under the lid. Such cases may require early lid surgery to correct the abnormal head position.

If there is an associated strabismus, eye muscle surgery to correct this problem is usually performed first, since the position of the lid may be affected by the eye position. Although eyelid surgery is quite effective, postoperative results are seldom perfect. In some cases the eyelid muscle is shortened (levator resection); in others, the lid must be suspended from the brow by transplanted connective tissue or by sutures. In general, it's much better to have a slight undercorrection than to have the lid elevated so much that it doesn't close normally, which could lead to problems from drying of the cornea.

Ptosis in itself hardly ever causes loss of vision, though amblyopia can result because children with ptosis are more likely than other children to have refractive errors. An eye doctor should examine any child with ptosis during the first year or so, to avoid the development of amblyopia.

Hemangiomas

Hemangiomas are benign tumors of the blood vessels that can occur anywhere in the body. They are more common in girls than in boys. In most cases they begin several weeks after birth as reddish or purple "bumps" on the skin. Their growth may be rapid for the first several months or even longer. Some are very small, a fraction of an inch in

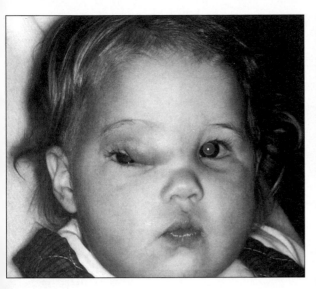

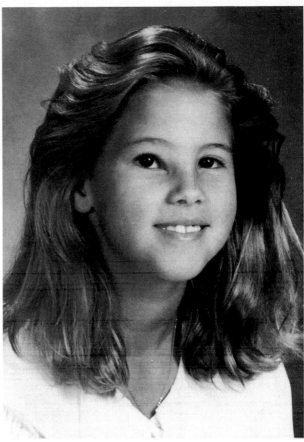

HEMANGIOMA . Above: A large hemangioma in the nasal portion of the right upper lid compresses the eye, causing astigmatism and amblyopia. Right: The same patient 11 years later with nearly complete resolution of the tumor, but with poor vision in the right eye.

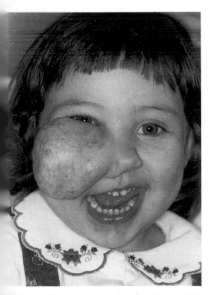

A large hemangioma in another child, now being treated for amblyoopia.

diameter, and others can be so large that they involve half the infant's head.

Typically the size remains the same for several years, and then gradually decreases so that even a large hemangioma is usually hard to detect by the teenage years. Of course there are exceptions, and some parents are disappointed that they don't disappear completely.

A hemangioma on the eyelid can affect an infant's vision by causing severe amblyopia. This can happen if the tumor is so large that it covers the pupil and obstructs vision (in much the same way that a cataract does). Or the mass may push on the soft infant eye, distorting its optics. It is common to find extreme degrees of astigmatism in such cases.

Treatment with glasses and patching may help. Sometimes the growth can be reversed with steroids, which may be taken orally, injected into the hemangioma under general anesthesia, or used topically as an ointment. But steroids can have side effects, so most ophthalmologists prefer not to use them unless the child's vision is threatened. Surgery to remove the hemangioma is reserved for severe cases.

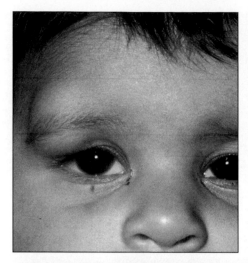

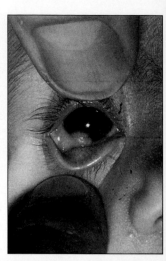

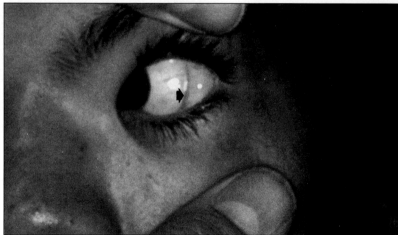

THREE KINDS OF DERMOID:

Upper left. This relatively large orbital dermoid is in the most common location, at the temporal end of the brow. It should be removed so that it does not rupture.

Upper right. A limbal dermoid may require partial excision during childhood because of its cosmetic impact.

Bottom. A lipodermoid, in this case in the temporal conjuntiva (arrow), is usually observed without surgery.

Dermoids

Dermoids are benign growths of unknown cause that contain elements normally found in the skin. A dermoid can occur in other parts of the body, but is commonly found around and on the eyes. A dermoid does not interfere with vision and is usually only a cosmetic problem.

One type appears as a painless pea- or marble-sized lump beneath the skin, typically at the outer margin of the eyebrow. It may grow slowly in the first few years of life. Other types of dermoid present as flesh-colored masses on the surface of the eye. They may extend onto the cornea or may hide as a barely apparent fold in the conjunctiva at the corner of the eye.

Appropriate treatment depends on location and symptoms. If it is considered unacceptably unsightly, a dermoid can be removed with elective surgery. An orbital dermoid should probably be removed lest it rupture and cause inflammation.

Corneal clouding

Opacification of the cornea in infancy has the same effect as a cataract: it can cause severe amblyopia. The problem appears in one or both eyes as a haze or whitening in front of the pupil (a cataract is behind the pupil). The most common cause is glaucoma, which also causes light sensitivity. In other cases there may be a metabolic disease, which may run in the family and may affect other parts of the body. Examples include the mucopolysaccharidoses and familial dysautonomia (Riley-Day syndrome). Clouding can also result from damage to the cornea by infection or trauma. In some children the cornea is improperly formed and cannot remain clear. Peter syndrome is described in Chapter 13.

The appropriate treatment depends on the cause and the severity of the opacification. Glaucoma requires urgent medical and surgical treatment. Both bacterial and viral infections can be treated medically, as can some metabolic diseases. Sometimes a contact lens can improve the optics. But in severe cases, corneal transplantation is required. In this surgical procedure, the cloudy cornea is cut away and replaced by a donor cornea. Although it is difficult to perform such surgery in young children, it may be the only way to achieve useful vision.

Uveitis

The middle layer of the eye, which is made up of the iris, the ciliary body and the choroid, is collectively called the *uvea*; its inflammation is called *uveitis*, and it can happen at any age. The symptoms depend on which part of the eye is affected. In the front of the eye, uveitis may cause redness, discomfort, and light sensitivity. Uveitis may be called *iritis* if the iris is affected. In the back of the eye, uveitis often causes no discomfort. In either place it can result in loss of vision. Ironically, those cases with fewer symptoms may have a more dangerous course because, among other reasons, they are detected less quickly.

Many parasitic, bacterial and viral infections can cause uveitis in children. Toxoplasmosis, for example, is a parasitic disease that can be acquired by a pregnant woman from cat litter or uncooked meat and then passed on to her baby before birth.

Most cases of uveitis are not infectious, and in most the cause is never known. Children with inflammatory diseases elsewhere in the body—arthritis or colitis, for example—may be prone to develop uveitis as well. The association is especially important in the case of juvenile rheumatoid arthritis. Children with this disease should see an ophthalmologist several times a year, especially if their blood tests are positive for antinuclear antibodies and negative for rheuma-

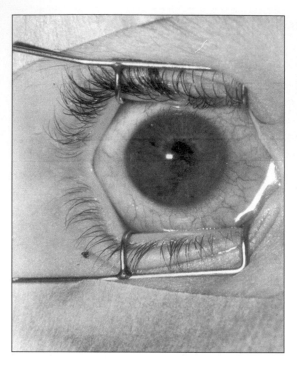

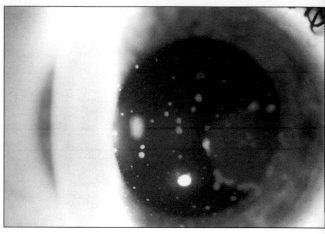

UVEITIS
Left. Inflammatory debris clouds the anterior chamber.

Right. A highly magnified view of another eye shows inflammatory deposits on the back of the cornea.

toid factor. Girls with only a few involved joints are especially at risk of uveitis.

The treatment depends on the cause. Infections can be treated with specific anti-infective medications. Even when the cause is not known, treatment of the inflammation itself can be highly effective. Steroid medications can be given by means of eyedrops or eye ointment, by injection next to the eye, or by mouth. Eyedrops are commonly used to keep the pupil dilated and help control the inflammation, especially for iritis.

Uveitis sometimes responds to treatment and lasts just a short time, or, in spite of excellent treatment, it may be chronic and unremitting. Severe cases can lead to glaucoma, cataracts, or damage to the cornea, retina and optic nerve.

Dislocation of the lens

The lens is suspended directly behind the center of the pupil by the zonules. If some of the zonules are broken, the lens may dislocate, so that only part of it remains behind the pupil, it becomes tilted, or it falls away from the pupil altogether. Parents may notice a wiggling move-

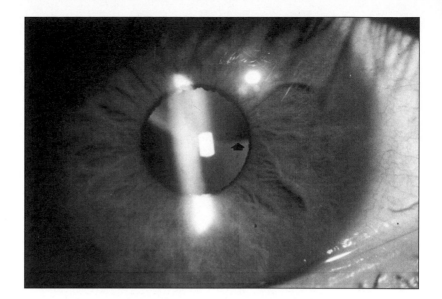

DISLOCATED LENS. The lens has dislocated upward, so that its lower edge is visible in the pupil from 3:00 to 10:00 (arrow). The vertical white band is the light from the slit lamp.

ment (called *iridodonesis)*, which results when the iris is not normally supported by the lens.

One cause of a dislocated lens is *Marfan syndrome*, which is acquired as an autosomal dominant trait (its other manifestations are long arms and legs, lax joints and heart problems). Another is *homocystinuria*, a disorder that shares some characteristics with Marfan except that it is autosomal recessive. Trauma to the eye is a common cause in older children. In many cases there is no apparent cause for the dislocated lens and there is no associated systemic disease.

Treatment can be difficult. Vitamin B6 or dietary therapy may be helpful in some cases of homocystinuria. If the dislocation is mild, glasses can correct the resulting nearsightedness and astigmatism. If it is possible for the child to see around the edge of the lens, the visual acuity might be better, but glasses or contact lenses for far-sightedness will be needed.

If the dislocation disrupts the eye's optics severely, the lens may need to be surgically removed. This surgery is the same as that used to remove a cataract. Similarly, surgery may be necessary if the lens falls through the pupil into the anterior chamber of the eye, though some ophthalmologists prefer to treat this condition medically by dilating the pupil to reposition the lens. If the lens dislocates into the vitreous, it can usually be left alone without any ill effect, though, again, optical correction will be needed.

Retinoblastoma

Retinoblastoma is a malignant eye tumor that not only can destroy a child's vision, but can be fatal as well. One or both eyes may be affected. The tumor usually appears in the first year or two of life as white reflection in the pupil, an appearance referred to as *leukocoria* (literally, "white pupil"). It may cause strabismus. Since it is often hereditary, babies who are close relatives of people with retinoblastoma should be examined soon after birth. If either parent has had a hereditary form of the disease, the risk for each child is 50%. The risk is lower if more distant relatives have been affected; blood tests can now help identify children who are likely to get the disease before the tumor can be seen.

Retinoblastoma is one of the most treatable of all childhood cancers. Although it is almost always fatal without treatment, it is rarely fatal with treatment. An eye with a very advanced tumor must be removed. Smaller tumors can be treated with radiation or chemother-

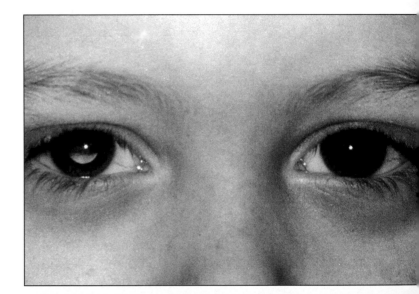

LEUKOCORIA FROM RETINOBLASTOMA

In the right eye, part of the pupil is white; compare to the normally black left pupil.

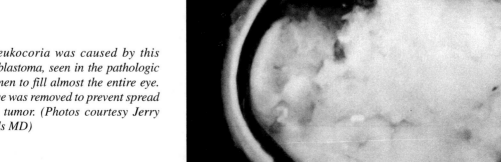

The leukocoria was caused by this retinoblastoma, seen in the pathologic specimen to fill almost the entire eye. The eye was removed to prevent spread of the tumor. (Photos courtesy Jerry Shields MD)

apy, and/or destroyed with laser or cryotherapy (freezing). If both eyes are involved, special efforts are made to save at least one eye.

If it is suspected that the malignancy has spread to other parts of the body, chemotherapy may be given. Even in children apparently cured of the disease, there is a tendency to develop other kinds of cancer, so close follow-up is important.

Colobomas

Long before birth, the developing eyeball is formed by the joining together of two edges of tissue, much like the two halves of a zipper. If a part of that "zipper" fails to close properly, a defect called a *colobo-*

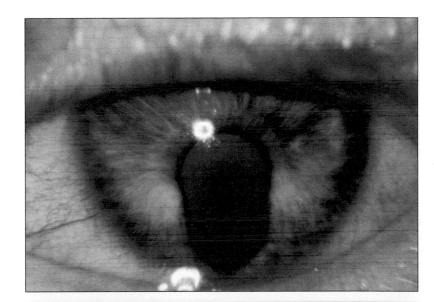

COLOBOMAS

A typical iris coloboma causes a vertically oval pupil.

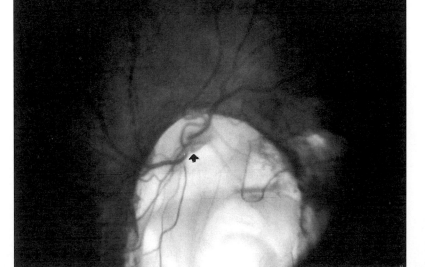

The coloboma in this case involves the optic nerve (arrow) and retina.

ma results, usually in the lower portion of the eye. The exact part of the eye involved depends upon what portion of the "zipper" fails to zip. Either one or both eyes may be affected.

When the coloboma occurs in the iris, a notch may be seen in the pupil. A child with this condition is sometimes said to have a "cat's eye" pupil. Farther back in the eye, a coloboma may affect the retina or the choroid, where it can be seen inside the eye as a whitish area of exposed sclera. A coloboma may also involve the optic nerve. An eye with a coloboma in any location may be smaller than normal, which is an additional indication that the eye did not form quite normally.

How badly the vision is impaired and what treatment is given depend on where the coloboma is located and what complications result from it. Every child with an abnormal pupil should have a careful examination to look for other colobomas. The child may need glasses, as well as patching for amblyopia. A special contact lens can be designed to cover a notched pupil to improve the eye's appearance, though the notch by itself causes no loss of vision. Sometimes a retinal coloboma is associated with a retinal hole or detachment that requires surgical repair. If a coloboma affects the optic nerve, the child's visual acuity will be at least mildly impaired. If the central part of the retina (the macula) is involved by the coloboma, the vision loss is usually severe.

Retinopathy of prematurity

The blood vessels that supply the peripheral portions of the retina are among the last parts of the eye to develop before birth. If the baby is born prematurely, these vessels may still be developing, not having reached the far periphery of the retina. This portion of the retina, especially on the side away from the nose, may be inadequately supplied with blood *(ischemia)*.

After birth, the growth of new abnormal vessels on and in front of the retina may be stimulated, potentially damaging the retina. This disease is called *retinopathy of prematurity* (ROP). Children who are most likely to be affected are those with very low birth weights (less than 1,500 grams, or about three pounds), those who are born very early, and those who require oxygen in high doses for a long time.

Fortunately, most cases resolve with relatively little damage. Careful eye examinations in the nursery are recommended. If damage is severe, freezing or laser treatments can often prevent further damage by stopping the growth of these abnormal vessels. But sometimes the process continues even with treatment, and the retina gets pulled away from its normal position inside the eye; this is called a *retinal detachment*. All children with ROP should be checked after several months to see whether they need glasses, since many are nearsighted. They also have an increased risk of strabismus and amblyopia.

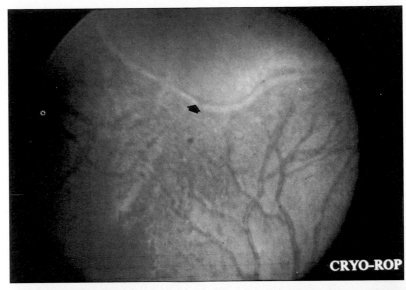

RETINOPATHY OF PREMATURITY

The ridge from 11:00 to 2:00 (arrow) marks the border between normally vascularized retina below and ischemic retina above. New, abnormal blood vessels may grow in this area and damage the retina.

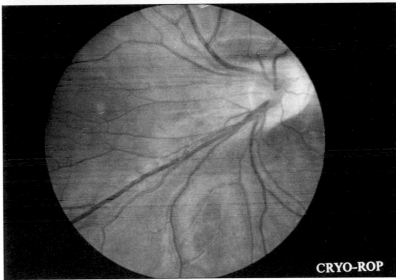

Traction in the retina is caused by the new blood vessels. It can result in loss of vision from distortion of the macula or, in severe cases, from retinal detachment. Compare with normal eye, page 19. (Photos from the Cryo-ROP Study courtesy Earl Palmer, MD).

Leber's congenital amaurosis

Children who have *Leber's congenital amaurosis* are nearly blind at birth because the photoreceptors (rods and cones) don't function. Nystagmus develops in the first several months of life. There is no treatment to improve their vision.

This is a very rare congenital condition of unknown cause. It can be diagnosed with a test called an *electroretinogram* (ERG), which measures the electrical impulses in the eye. Leber's is hereditary (autosomal recessive); if one child is affected, there is one chance in four that each child of the same parents will have the disease. Unfortunately, at this time there is no way to tell whether a fetus will be affected. But that may soon change because of rapid advances in molecular genetics. Children with Leber's usually have normal intelligence and can benefit from programs designed to help children adjust to impaired vision and lead productive lives.

Color blindness

True color "blindness" *(achromatopsia)* is quite rare. But about one out of every 17 males has abnormal color perception. They are said to be color blind, but this is a misnomer. Men and boys with this problem can see colors, but they need brighter shades to distinguish reds from greens (the colors most commonly confused) or yellows from blues. Visual acuity is completely normal. Because this condition is inherited as a sex-linked, recessive trait, unaffected mothers pass it to their sons, half of whom will be affected. Girls rarely have the disorder.

Children who are color blind hardly ever have trouble learning their colors. But teachers who use color-coded educational materials need to be aware of the problem. Color-blind people may have to avoid certain careers in which the ability to make subtle color distinctions is crucial, and they occasionally need help picking two socks that match. But they usually can drive without difficulty and most are rarely troubled by their problem.

Optic nerve hypoplasia

If the optic nerve is improperly formed before birth, it may be small in size, pale in color, or misshapen in contour. This improper formation, called *optic nerve hypoplasia,* can affect one or both eyes and can vary from barely detectable to extremely severe. The optic nerve carries the visual information from the retina to the brain, and if the defect is severe, it may cause the eye to see poorly. In bilateral cases, it may induce nystagmus. The visual outcome for a child with this condition can range from nearly normal vision to complete blindness. The disease does not worsen over time.

Because the optic nerve is part of the brain, it is not surprising that optic nerve hypoplasia is sometimes associated with other developmental abnormalities. Septo-optic dysplasia (DeMorsier's syndrome) includes agenesis of the corpus collosum and the septum pellucidum. Many times these structural defects in the brain are of little significance. But sometimes they can affect the functioning of the pituitary gland. X-ray and endocrine evaluations are therefore important for any child with optic nerve hypoplasia who experiences a delay in growth.

OPTIC NERVE HYPOPLASIA

In the right eye, the retinal vessels emanate from a small and pale optic nerve (smaller arrow) which is surrounded by a pigmented ring. The outer white ring (larger arrow) is the sclera adjacent to the optic nerve.

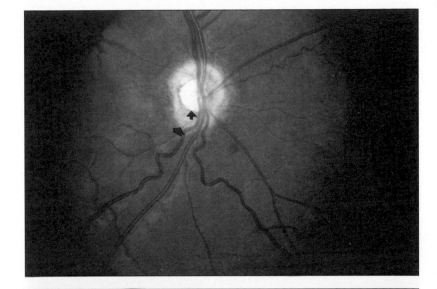

The optic nerve in the left eye of this child is normal.

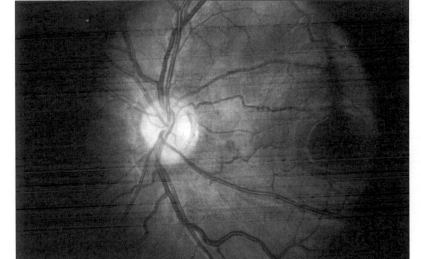

Optic atrophy and papilledema

The healthy optic nerve is pinkish-yellow where it enters the eye. If the nerve is pale, when viewed through the pupil with an ophthalmoscope, it indicates that it is damaged in some way. That condition is called *optic nerve atrophy* or *optic atrophy*. Because the optic nerve transmits visual information from the retina to the brain, optic atrophy usually causes some degree of visual loss. That visual loss may include a loss of color perception, a loss of peripheral vision, or a loss of central vision. Usually there is some combination of all three.

Optic nerve atrophy may have various underlying causes, including tumors in the brain or in the orbit. It may be hereditary (autosomal dominant), or it may result from a severe injury to the head or

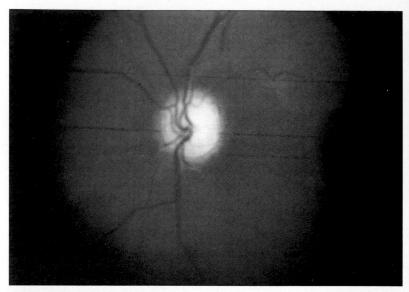

OPTIC ATROPHY. The normal pink-yellow color of the optic nerve is replaced by the pale, nearly white color of optic atrophy. Note the paucity of small blood vessels on the disc's surface.

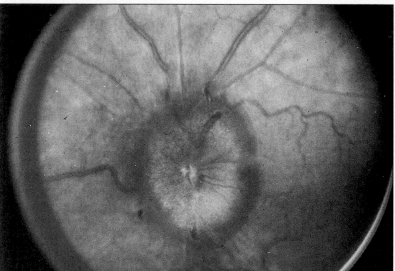

PAPILLEDEMA. In this case of florid papilledema, the disc is elevated, its margins are blurred, and the capillaries on its surface are dilated.

eye. The ophthalmologist will look for the cause of the optic atrophy and try to eliminate it if possible.

Examination of the optic nerve may indicate that something is wrong with the brain itself. If the pressure in the brain is too high—for example, because of a tumor—there may be *papilledema*, a swelling of the optic nerve. If this is discovered on eye examination, the ophthalmologist will likely suggest neuro-imaging. Depending on what is found, neurosurgical treatment may be appropriate.

Visual impairment due to cerebral palsy and other central nervous system disorders

Many children with cerebral palsy or other developmental or neurologic problems also seem to see poorly. At first they may show little interest in their visual environment, staring at the ground or into space rather than looking at faces or toys. They may not even respond when a bright light is directed at their eyes. Characteristically, though, their pupils react normally and they do not have nystagmus as might be expected in a child with a severe eye disorder. In fact, careful examination of the eyes usually shows that they are practically normal.

The problem, of course, is in the visual areas of the brain. Just as other neurologic problems may improve over time, visual responsiveness may improve as well, but the rate and extent are hard to predict. A few children never seem to get better. It is important for parents to realize that even these children may actually "see" better than they appear to demonstrate to those around them. All children with these disorders should be given the benefit of normal visual environment, with mobiles over their cribs and other visually attractive toys, even though the hoped-for improvement in visual behavior has not yet occurred.

19

Eye Injuries

Ellen was only six years old, and she didn't see any reason not to pick up the cuddly little puppy who lived next door. Unfortunately, its mother was displeased and, without warning, jumped at Ellen and bit her in the eyelid. Blood was everywhere.

Three-year-old Jennifer was playing with her little brother near the wood stove. The ashes were cool—so cool, in fact, that they felt good between her fingers. She discovered it was fun to toss the fine powder into the air, letting it fall on her face. Her mother, busy in the next room, didn't know what the children were doing. But suddenly Jennifer ran to her screaming. Her left eye was firery red, tearing, and swollen shut. Jennifer's mother immediately took her to the hospital. When the doctor opened her eye, part of the cornea was white.

Five-year-old John and his friend Ken were playing catch with an old tennis ball. Somehow John just wasn't looking when the ball bounced up and hit his left eye really hard. He cried from the pain. Then he realized he couldn't see normally with that eye and became absolutely terrified. His vision was getting worse every second. He was sure that he was going blind. He wondered what it would be like to learn Braille. After a few minutes, he fell asleep.

Brad, age four, was in the back yard riding his tricycle. His dad was in the garage, just a few steps away. Suddenly Brad cried out in pain. His right eye was full of blood, and there was a large laceration *through the cornea. X-rays showed a BB in the right eye, just behind the lens. After five hours of emergency surgery, Brad's eye was saved, but his vision will never be normal.*

～

Accidents in which children's eyes are injured are usually freak occurrences, certainly never predictable. And they are always frightening to both the child and the parents. One of us (JWS) will never forget the feelings he had when he was hit in the eye with that tennis ball at age 5. And we both have kids ourselves, so we can understand the terror parents endure when their children are in the emergency department or operating room because of a serious eye injury.

Unfortunately, such accidents happen all too often. Each year in the United States there are more than two million eye injuries severe enough to require medical attention or decreased activity. Because most blinding injuries strike children and young adults, they cause disproportionate impact in terms of years of disability. More than half of the eyes lost in children are lost as the result of injury.

Although some types of injuries take place during dangerous play, many do not. We've seen eyes lost because a child fell against a shrub, because another child threw a ballpoint pen in a classroom, or because an exercise machine broke. Many eyes are injured in fights. And it's sad to say, but many children also suffer serious eye injuries because of child abuse. Certainly these are preventable, and so are most of the others.

Initial evaluation and first aid

A parent's immediate response when a child sustains an eye injury is to panic. Even to the doctor it may seem critical to "do something" immediately. To be sure, seconds can count if a caustic chemical is splashed in an eye. But no other kind of eye injury demands immediate treatment, and there's ample time to get the child to the hospital for a careful and thorough examination, under anesthesia in the operating room if necessary.

Seconds count if a caustic chemical is splashed in an eye. No other kind of eye injury demands immediate treatment.

Trauma is one of the most unpredictable eye problems, and serious injuries can be inapparent at first. So, before going too far with definitive treatment, or even with predicting a return of vision, an ophthalmologist needs to take the necessary time—sometimes even days or weeks—to evaluate the damage carefully.

Some eye injuries, for instance those resulting from falls or motor vehicle accidents, can be accompanied by other serious trauma. Ex-

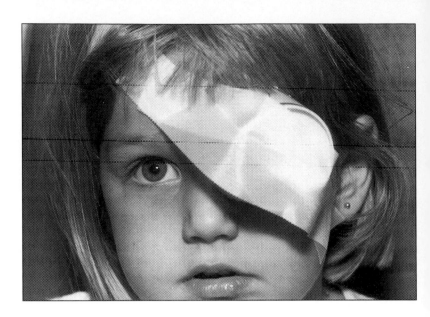

PROTECTIVE SHIELD FOR AN INJURED EYE. Temporary first aid for a seriously injured eye might include a shield fashioned from a paper cup which can be taped over the eye to prevent further damage.

amination and treatment of the eye must wait until the child has been stabilized and any life-threatening injuries have been treated. In the meantime, the goal is to protect the injured eye. If the eye is lacerated, a protective patch or shield should be taped over it so that no pressure will be placed on the eye that might cause further damage. For the same reason, it is best for injured children to lie on their back and avoid coughing or other types of straining.

Examination and history   Sometimes the circumstances of an injury can provide a clue to the kind of damage an eye has suffered. Striking two pieces of metal together may dislodge a shard with sufficient force to penetrate an eye and yet cause very little pain or redness. An injury involving sharp, pointed objects such as darts or knives can cause deep injuries to the eye, the orbit, and even the brain, all with little outside evidence.

A recurring problem with injuries in children is that there may be no reliable way of finding out what happened. Sometimes no adult was present and the child is too young to give the doctor an accurate history. Other times children are afraid to tell the truth because the injury happened when they were doing something they know they weren't supposed to. All children with histories suspicious of child abuse should be examined by an ophthalmologist, since retinal hemorrhages are a key finding in "shaken baby" injuries.

Examination in the emergency department should be as complete as possible and should include a measurement of visual acuity. However, detailed examination may be impossible at first, as struggling with a frightened child is often not fruitful and could even lead to further damage. Clues to damage inside the eye may be suggested by the abnormal size, shape, or reactivity of the affected pupil or by a reduction of the pressure or volume inside the eye. Abnormal eye movements may signify a problem in the eye, the orbit, or even the brain. Whenever more than the most insignificant injury is suspected, an ophthalmologist should be consulted.

Trauma to the front of the eye may be apparent only on microscopic examination. Damage to the retina or the vitreous can often be seen through the dilated pupil using an ophthalmoscope. X-rays, neuro-imaging techniques, and ultrasound are particularly useful when a foreign body or some form of damage inside or behind the eye is suspected. When a serious eye injury is suspected in a child,

When a serious eye injury is suspected in a child, a complete eye exam is usually deferred until the child is under general anesthesia.

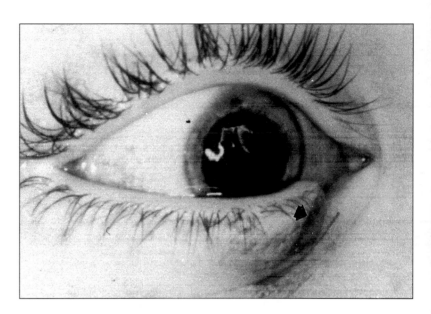

LACERATION OF THE LOWER CANALICULUS

This eyelid laceration (arrow) extends downward from the margin across the area where the inferior canaliculus passes.

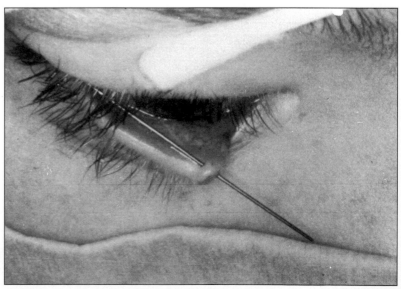

A probe inserted through the lower punctum exits through the wound, confirming the laceration of the canaliculus. Abnormal tearing can be expected if the canaliculus is not repaired. (Photo courtesy Dale Meyer, MD)

a complete eye exam is usually deferred until the child is under general anesthesia.

External injuries

Laceration of the eyelids or tear ducts   After the puppy bit Ellen's eyelid *(story, page 168)*, it bled so much that her mother couldn't tell how bad the injury was. She was terrified.

Ellen was fortunate in that her injury, like most lid injuries, was not serious. An eyelid laceration can be sutured like a laceration anywhere else and it will heal rapidly. But eyelids are a very cosmetically sensitive area, so the suturing should be done by someone with exper-

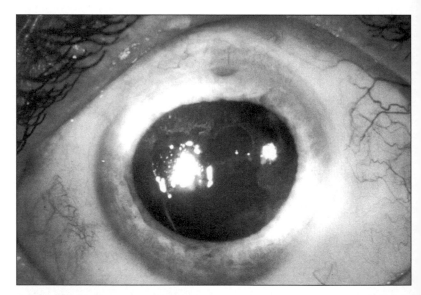

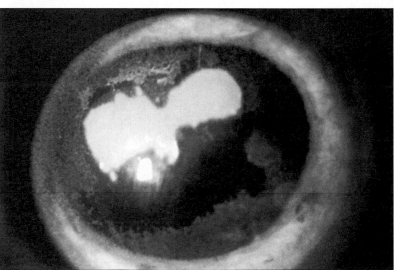

CORNEAL ABRASION. Top: A large corneal abrasion is better seen after fluorescein is instilled (bottom), partially staining the abraded cornea.

ience. Problems are especially likely when the cut goes across the lid margin, since imprecise repair can cause unattractive notching.

If the eyelid margin has been cut, an ophthalmologist should be called in to repair the lid under general anesthesia. Even more delicate is the suturing needed to fix a cut through the tear duct. This can take hours of work using an operating microscope. *Most important, the evaluation of any eyelid injury should include a careful examination to make sure that the eye has not also been damaged.*

Corneal abrasion   Probably the most common eye injury seen in an emergency department is abrasion of the cornea. Something scratching the very sensitive surface of the cornea will cause severe discomfort along with tearing and redness of the eye. An abrasion can be caused by almost anything: a fingernail, a pillowcase, a contact lens, even a lighted cigarette. The outline of the abrasion can be seen using fluorescein, a very useful orange dye that can be placed in the tears. It fills the abrasion and glows when viewed in blue light.

A mild abrasion will heal in a day or two. During that time the child may be more comfortable with a patch taped on tightly so the lids don't rub across the sore eye with each blink. Usually an antibiotic drop or ointment is placed in the eye to prevent infection. Very rarely, there is a problem with healing. Spontaneous recurrences, called *recurrent erosions*, are a possible complication.

Foreign bodies   At one time or another, nearly all children manage to get a foreign body in one of their eyes. It usually comes out by itself, helped along by a flood of tears. Sometimes, though, a foreign body will stick to the surface of the cornea. It's usually tiny,

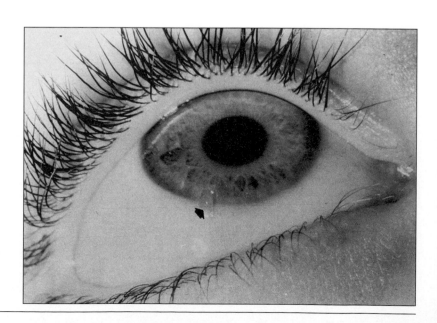

CORNEAL FOREIGN BODY. This relatively large, apparently organic foreign body has lodged at the 7:00 limbus (arrow).

but you can almost always see a speck if you look very closely. Occasionally the foreign body will work its way under the upper lid and stick to the inside surface. That's an unfortunate resting place: with each blink the nasty thing scratches the cornea.

The treatment is, of course, to remove the foreign object. Sometimes you can get it out with a moistened cotton-tipped swab. In a young child it may be necessary for an ophthalmologist to remove it from the cornea using a tiny needle under anesthesia. (Obviously it's dangerous to use anything sharp near the eye unless the child is certain to be very still.)

Unless it is very deep, a foreign body on the cornea usually causes little trouble if it's appropriately treated. Sometimes a metallic object will leave a *rust ring* embedded in the superficial cornea even after it has been removed; the rust ring can be taken out later or even left in place. As with corneal abrasions, using an antibiotic drop or ointment and patching the eye for a day or two after removal may be helpful.

Chemical burns

The ashes that fell into Jennifer's eye *(story, page 168)* caused a chemical burn from the extremely strong alkali (lye) they contain. Acids can be almost as harmful. Both chemicals damage the cornea, in severe cases causing it to lose its clarity. The conjunctiva can also be damaged, leading to scarring and loss of normal tear production. This damage makes it difficult to replace the cornea later with a transplant. Alkali can even penetrate to the inside of the eye, causing a cataract or glaucoma.

The severity of a chemical burn depends on how strong the acid or alkali is and how much has entered the eye. But it also depends

ALKALI DAMAGE TO THE CORNEA. A strong alkali can seriously damage the cornea and cause it to become opaque. Note the eye appears white and comfortable because blood vessels in the conjunctiva and sensory nerves in the cornea have been destroyed.

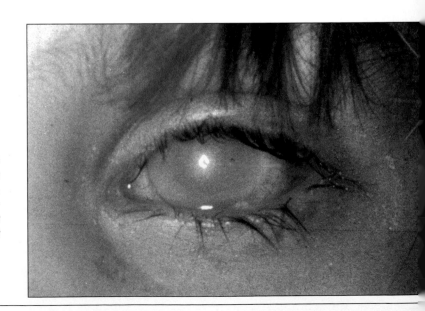

on how long the chemical is allowed to remain there. Normal reflexes help. First, the eyes are flooded with tears, which dilute and wash the chemical away. Second, most people instinctively rush to find water. This is when seconds can count. Ophthalmologists recommend washing out the open eye continuously for a half hour or more using as much as a liter or two of water. It is a good idea for parents to help children wash out their eyes if they get anything into them that stings, and to keep washing them out, meanwhile calling for help.

Later treatment should be prescribed by an ophthalmologist, and may include the use of local antibiotics, steroid drops to control inflammation, and medications to control a destructive enzyme *(collagenase)* that is released following injury.

Blunt injuries

The bones of the orbital rim are a fairly effective barrier against objects larger than about 4 inches across. A large object could break these bones if they were struck hard enough, but it's usually a smaller object —a ball, the end of a bat, a hockey puck or a fist, for example—that causes injury to the eye itself. The sudden compression (the "shock wave," so to speak) from a blunt injury can damage nearly every part of the eye, even though the eyeball is not penetrated.

John was hit in the eye with a tennis ball. His story *(page 168)* is fairly typical of how a child can receive a blunt injury to the eye. John had the usual components of a blunt injury: his lids were bruised and there was blood under the conjunctiva. Although impressive to look at, these injuries are not usually serious. More important was the bleeding inside the eye, called a *hyphema.* The blood occupies

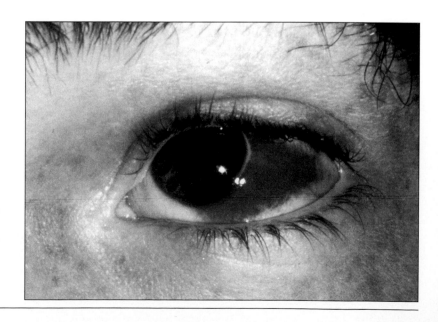

SUBCONJUNCTIVAL HEMORRHAGE. Blood under the conjunctiva may result from blunt trauma. It is not itself dangerous, but there may be significant associated injury.

HYPHEMA. Blood in the anterior chamber has partially clotted, obscuring the iris inferiorly.

the anterior chamber (between the cornea and the iris), and vision usually becomes poor because blood blocks light from entering the pupil. In most cases the blood will clear without complication, but bleeding can recur during the first few days after the trauma. To prevent this, most ophthalmologists like to have children curtail their activities, and sometimes both eyes are patched to discourage eye movement. It may be a protective reflex for children to get sleepy, as happened to John.

A blunt injury can cause other problems as well.

o Glaucoma may develop, either at the time of the injury or up

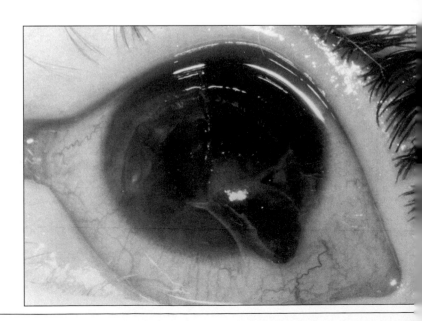

RUPTURED EYE. Blunt trauma of sufficient force may rupture the cornea or sclera. In this case, a knuckle of iris has come forward and has prolapsed through the corneal wound.

to many years later. Anyone who has had a hyphema should probably be checked for glaucoma every year or so.

o Inflammation inside the eye, called *iritis*, may be associated. Affected children will be sensitive to light.

o The lens may be knocked out of position (dislocated) or a cataract may develop.

o There may be blood in the vitreous, perhaps obscuring vision for months.

o The retina may be torn, causing a retinal detachment or other damage.

o The eye, if struck with sufficient force, may even rupture.

The treatment of a blunt injury and the visual prognosis depend on the extent of injury. Treatment may be urgent, since a damaged eye can become amblyopic during the weeks, or even days, that its vision is poor. Medications can help fight off infection, control inflammation and treat glaucoma. Surgery may be necessary if a hyphema doesn't clear and there are complications. Similarly, surgery may be needed to remove a cataract, repair a detached retina, or suture a ruptured eye.

Penetrating injuries

A penetrating injury is one in which an object actually goes into the eyeball. It may be caused by a fast-moving projectile such as a BB, piece of glass, or tiny sliver of metal, or by a sharp, pointed object such as a knife or dart. Around the Fourth of July we often see injuries of this type caused by fireworks.

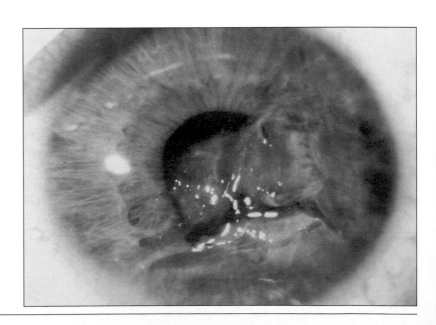

CORNEAL LACERATION. The corneal wound will require repair using very fine sutures, viewed with the magnification of an operating microscope. Because the stellate laceration crosses the pupillary axis, some loss of vision is inevitable.

As Brad's case *(story, page 168)* illustrates, a penetrating injury may be caused by something that remains inside the eye or behind it in the orbit. Although careful examination is critical, sometimes the foreign body can be found only by using such studies as CAT or MRI scans, x-rays with dental film, or ultrasonography.

The first step is to examine the eye to see just how bad the injury is. Unfortunately, it's often worse than initially expected. With the child under anesthesia, the ophthalmologist can clean and carefully probe the wound.

If surgery is needed it will usually be performed during the same anesthesia. Blood and other debris may be removed, and wounds in the cornea or the sclera repaired with fine sutures. If there is a foreign body inside the eye or the orbit, it will probably be removed. Metals, especially, can damage the retina or cause glaucoma, and many substances can cause harmful inflammation. Removing an object from the inside of the eye or the orbit is always difficult, but it can be easier if the object is magnetic. Antibiotics are given before and after surgery.

In severe cases, repair of damage inside the eye may have to be delayed until the eye begins to heal. The interval between the surgeries will allow some of the blood to clear and changes in the vitreous to take place so that the second surgery will be more effective.

The amount of vision recovered following a serious injury is sometimes surprising. Even if vision is not fully restored, it is important to remember that any level of vision may be precious if the other eye ever fails.

But some cases don't turn out so well. If the patient cannot see even a bright light after a week or so, it is probably best that the eye be removed. A severely injured eye, if not taken out, occasionally sets up an inflammatory disease that can damage the good eye. Although

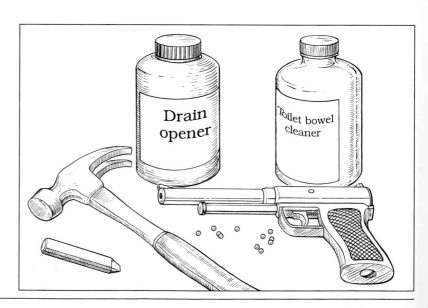

HAZARDOUS OBJECTS. Children should be supervised around all these, as each can cause serious eye injury.

this disease, called *sympathetic ophthalmitis*, is rare, preserving the injured eye is just not worth the risk if it has no vision at all.

Once an eye is removed and replaced with an artificial sphere, the child's appearance will be better. The lids will close over a smooth surface that looks like the inside of the lip. Later a painted plastic shell will be carefully crafted to match the other eye. This prosthesis can be left in place for weeks or months at a time. It can be removed as needed for cleaning with plain soap and water. Prostheses are now so well made that it is often hard to tell which of the patient's eyes is the real one and which is artificial.

Prevention

Young people should be appropriately supervised around pointed objects, BB guns, and pieces of metal that are struck together (such as a hammer and chisel). Small children should not have access to caustic chemicals, and people of all ages should take extra care when using such household products as drain openers and toilet-bowl cleaners. Children should never be allowed to play with fireworks unsupervised. And everyone should use seat belts or safety seats in cars and helmets when they're riding their bicycles.

One of the most important measures parents can take is to insist that their children wear appropriate protective eyewear. Sports goggles and headgear are available that, when properly worn, are effective even in games involving fast-moving objects and vigorous physical contact.

It's especially important for any child who has impaired vision in one eye to wear such protection. We'll always remember one child, blind in the right eye since birth, who was up at bat in a baseball game. He wasn't looking when the pitcher threw the baseball, and it hit him squarely in his good eye. Fortunately he was wearing his safety goggles. The goggles were broken, but the boy's eye was unharmed.

Children who rely on one good eye should take extra care to protect it. The American Academy of Ophthalmology recommends that they wear safety glasses full-time, even if they don't need glasses to correct their vision. (The glasses need not be ugly.) Parents should ask

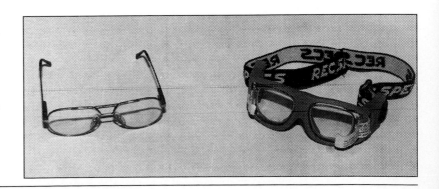

PROTECTIVE EYEWEAR. The pair of glasses on the left is made to meet the American National Standards Institute's Z.87 standard for eye protection. Even stronger are the sports goggles on the right. The American Academy of Ophthalmology recommends full-time eye protection for all who have good vision in only one eye.

their optician for a pair that meets the American National Standards Institute's specification for toughness (ANSI Z.87). And for all children, safety goggles are recommended for sports—such as squash, hockey and lacrosse—that involve small balls or sticks as standard equipment.

NON-MEDICAL
PROBLEMS

20 The Child with Impaired Vision

*J*oan and Marilyn were cousins who had practically grown up together. But they seemed to drift apart after Marilyn's first child, Jack, was born with an eye problem that made him "legally blind." Joan had wondered if Marilyn was embarrassed by his handicap.

It was not until Jack was four that the two women saw each other again, when Marilyn invited Joan to stop by. Joan observed Jack closely and was a bit surprised that he seemed so normal. He played with the neighborhood children, he rode his tricycle in the driveway, and he ran into the house occasionally to interrupt their conversation with some bit of information that just couldn't wait. Later when he came inside he sat close to the television, but Joan realized that her own children did the same thing. She couldn't understand how Jack could seem to see so well and yet be legally blind.

Some children do not see normally, even with the best doctors, glasses, medicines and surgery. Jack is one of them. Although no medical treatment can give him normal vision, much can be done to help him to make better use of the vision he does have and adapt in other ways to his visual disability.

Legal blindness does not necessarily mean that Jack is blind in the sense of not being able to see anything at all. It means that Jack's vision in his better eye (or with both eyes open), wearing the best possible glasses, is below a specific threshold.

The terms: legally blind, partially sighted, visually impaired, visually handicapped   The designation of legal blindness means that visual acuity is 20/200 or less, or that peripheral vision is less than 20°. Five out of every 10,000 American children fall into this category.

A much larger number of children are in the category termed *partially sighted*—those whose vision is better than 20/200 but poorer than 20/70. Such children may need some special help for specific school activities, but they are generally less impaired than those who are legally blind. The terms *visually impaired* and *visually handicapped*, which are synonyms, apply to both legally blind and partially sighted children.

How well does a legally blind child see?

Normal vision is 20/20. That means that at 20 feet the person can read very small figures on the Snellen eye chart. Some eyes see better than normal, say 20/15. At 20 feet a person with 20/15 vision can see the line on the chart that someone with normal vision could not see unless the chart were brought five feet closer.

A person with 20/200 vision—the threshold for legal blindness in most states—would see an object at 20 feet that the normal eye could see at 200 feet. Put another way, if Jack's vision is 20/200, he has to get much closer (in theory, 10 times as close) to see details that others with 20/20 vision can see.

Even though Jack is considered legally blind, there are many things he can see just fine. He sees large objects: the tree and the other children in the yard, cars that he rides his tricycle around, and large toys. He has to get close to see the leaves on the tree or facial features or the numbers on license plates, but at his age he doesn't need to see much detail. That's one reason Joan found his behavior normal; another is that he was in familiar territory and knew where most things were.

Some children who are legally blind do not see as well as Jack. They may be unable to see the big E at the top of the eye chart if their vision is worse than 20/400.

Testing for low vision   Children who cannot see the big E on the eye chart at 20 feet might have their vision tested at 10 or even 5 feet from the chart. If they cannot identify figures or letters at any distance, the doctor will test their vision by having them count fingers and noting how close they must be to see the fingers or their movements. If they cannot see well enough to identify hand movements, the examiner will test whether they can find, or even see, a bright light.

Loss of peripheral vision   So far we've described legal blindness as a loss of central vision, the inability to see things that are looked at directly. Often when central vision is poor, peripheral vision is relatively normal. Normal peripheral vision extends about 150° from one side to another. Because of the importance of peripheral vision, children who have visual fields of less than 20° are considered legally blind even when their central vision is 20/20. Such children see clearly, but it's as if they're looking down the barrel of a gun. They typically have trouble avoiding obstacles.

Parents' attitudes

The news that their child will have a permanent visual impairment can be devastating to parents. We all have a deep-seated dread of blindness, and it is often exaggerated by misconceptions. Parents may conjure up images of a helpless blind person struggling to get around with a white cane. And they may mistakenly blame themselves for the impairment.

Interestingly, the stages of adjustment to visual impairment may parallel those of adjustment to a terminal illness: rejection, "bargaining," anger, depression, and finally acceptance. Adjustment is more difficult if there are other impairments of if the child looks different from other children.

Parents' adjustment and adaptation to visual impairment are easier if they receive accurate information. They should learn their child's diagnosis, the possibility for medical treatment, the prognosis for improvement or worsening, and any other medical or genetic implications. Medical specialists can provide most of this information. Family support groups can be invaluable. In many cases, professional counseling is important for the whole family. Perhaps the most important realization is that, despite their obvious differences from children with normal vision, Jack and other children with visual impairments are more *like* other children than they are *unlike* them.

Early development

Children with Jack's degree of impairment are remarkably able to adapt, even from infancy, and they rarely seem to be handicapped in their activities at play or even at school through the early elementary years. They seem to reach their developmental milestones at the same ages as children with normal vision.

But children with more severely impaired vision—those who are unable to see figures at any distance—may have more trouble. After all, it is through vision that we put together most of what we know about our environment and learn to react to it from a very early age. Parents need to understand that their child who is unable to maintain eye contact or "smile back" is not rejecting them. They also need to understand that the child is not deaf just because he doesn't turn his face toward sounds; he may simply not know where the sounds are coming from.

People who have worked with children who have severely impaired vision know that many areas of development are affected. Reaching, crawling and walking are delayed simply because there is no visual enticement. Postural reflexes are affected early, and later children may have trouble with balance, especially when they're running or hopping. Because they cannot see the things around them, they may be slow to explore their environment. However, many people, even professionals, wrongly interpret the passivity of such children as stemming from a lack of intelligence rather than from under-stimulation.

Social development may be similarly delayed. Children will be less imaginative at play if they can't see who or what is available to play with. They will have trouble playing with construction toys, putting together puzzles, and drawing. As they encounter difficulty assessing their effect on others, they can become isolated and withdrawn. Later, they may have trouble understanding visually based concepts, such as colors and distances, and integrating related bits of information that their peers with normal vision can put together at a glance.

Ways to enhance development   From an early age, children with severe visual impairments may develop stereotypic patterns of behavior, such as gazing at lights, rocking, playing with their fingers in an exaggerated manner, or poking at their eyes. It is unclear why these behaviors develop, but they are common and do not necessarily indicate problems other than severely impaired vision.

Understanding these effects will enable parents to help their children compensate and cope. From the earliest age these children need to be stimulated through their other senses and through whatever vision they have. Their environment should be rich in colors, shapes, textures, sounds, and even tastes and smells. One helpful device is a chair with a tray that will allow objects to be explored up close both visually and by touch.

Older children have an easier time getting around their home if the furniture is left in the same place and if they can follow along walls and move from one object to the next. Without doubt, bringing up a child with severely impaired vision is more demanding for parents than bringing up a child with normal vision.

Outside resources   Help is available from many sources. The process of obtaining it usually begins with a referral to the local Association for the Blind, the State Commission for the Blind, or the low vision program in the local school district. Ophthalmologists, pediatricians, neurologists and other medical specialists provide diagnoses, medical and surgical treatment, and genetic counseling. Occupational therapists, psychologists, speech pathologists, educators, social workers and counselors each have their own perspectives and interventions and all can be immensely important to the child and the family.

Education

Until the end of the second world war, children with impaired vision were educated in boarding schools called sight conservation schools which operated on the false premise that what little sight they had was a limited resource that shouldn't be used excessively. Educational methods emphasized nonvisual learning. Children were taught Braille even when they had enough sight to read. Sixty years ago, Jack might have been discouraged from going to college, regardless of his intellect or ambition.

Fortunately, society has a much more enlightened approach today, as reflected by the landmark Education of All Handicapped Children Act, which became federal law in 1975. Only children with the most severe multiple disabilities now attend separate schools.

The vast majority of children with impaired vision attend regular public schools. In some large school districts they be taught by certified teachers of the visually impaired (TVIs) in separate classes. Other schools include a resource room, perhaps supervised by a TVI, where children spend part of each day, though most of the day they attend regular classes with normally sighted children. Itinerant programs are a third possibility. In these, children spend almost all the time in regular classes , but they have the services of a TVI several hours each week (the TVI may travel to several schools to provide services as needed).

The importance of educational evaluation   Several months before the placement of a child with impaired vision, a thorough educational evaluation must be performed. School personnel review records from the child's ophthalmologist, psychological and developmental assessments, speech and language evaluations, and other consultations. All this input will be considered in the development of a plan that describes the specific educational goals for the child based on individual abilities and needs.

The child's parents are included in this process and have specific rights. They should be prepared to act as advocates for their child. One important step is to make certain that evaluations are performed by professionals who are used to working with visually impaired children. Otherwise the child might be placed in an inappropriate school environment.

What a good educational program can provide   A key question in planning an education program is whether the impairment will prevent the child from learning to read the printed word easily.

When the answer is yes, the child will probably need to learn Braille. Textbooks will be "read" with the fingers and, for writing, a Braille stylus will be used to punch dots into a sheet of paper. The child's listening skills will be emphasized and developed at school, and talking books may use "compressed speech" to save time. The child will also be taught a variety of daily living skills to foster independence in dressing and, as as the years pass, handling money, shopping, cooking, using the telephone, and so on. Orientation and mobility instruction will allow the child to move around independently using a sighted guide or a cane, if needed.

For children like Jack, whose vision and developmental status permit the use of written words as the primary channel of learning, educational programming is much different. Jack will not need Braille at all, and he will have less need to be taught daily living skills or to receive orientation and mobility training. He'll spend almost all of his time in a regular class, either sitting in the front row or walking up to the board from time to time to get a closer look. An aide or his itinerant TVI may darken the words on his hand-outs, and his classroom teacher may give him extra time to read some assignments. Large-print books and magnifying devices may also help.

Availability of low vision aids   A variety of technological devices can help children with severely impaired vision to use whatever vision they have or to cope better without vision. Low vision aids are usually prescribed by eye doctors who specialize in low vision.

For older children, usually those past elementary school age, various types of telescopes (mounted onto glasses or held by hand) can help them see the blackboard, and magnifying lenses can help for reading. A closed circuit television (CCTV) can magnify printed materials and project them onto the screen, and allow the child to increase or decrease image size by turning a knob. A hand-held optical scanner passed across a page can reproduce the printing as a tactile array in which the letters can actually be felt or read out loud by a computer. Similar devices can print an image in any size desired. A computer program can read printed material and transcribe it into Braille, or translate Braille into print. Talking calculators, computers, and other aids are opening more doors of communication for children with even the most severely impaired vision.

No matter how mild or how severely impaired the vision, it's important for parents to enhance their children's self-esteem by concentrating on the child's strengths and abilities and perhaps encouraging them to develop a special talent. In all cases, they should be viewed as whole people. Impaired vision may require adaptation, but it should never be allowed to define the people who have it.

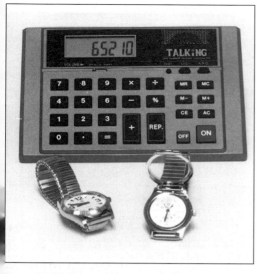

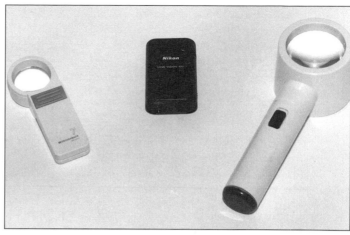

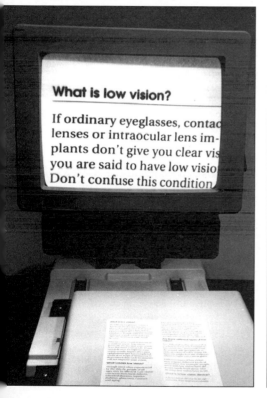

The six dots of the Braille cell are arranged and numbered

```
1 ● ● 4
2 ● ● 5
3 ● ● 6
```

● = raised
○ = smooth

| a | b | c | d | e | f | g | h |

The capital sign, dot 6, placed before a letter makes a capital letter

```
1   4
2   5
3 ● 6
```

The number sign, dots 3, 4, 5, 6, placed before the characters a through j, makes the numbers 1 through 0. For example: "a" preceded by the number sign is 1, "b" is 2, etc.

LOW VISION AIDS AND OTHER AIDS FOR THE VISUALLY IMPAIRED. Above, left: The talking calculator can be used by people unable to see the figures. The watch on the left has large numbers; the one on the right can be "read" with the fingers. Above, right: Various hand-held magnifying devices can be helpful for reading or distance viewing, and are sometimes mounted in spectacles. Below, left: Closed circuit TV can greatly magnify text. Below, right: The raised dots of the Braille alphabet are "read" with the fingers of those whose sight is too poor to read the printed word easily.

RESOURCES FOR CHILDREN WITH IMPAIRED VISION

1. American Association for Pediatric
    Ophthalmology and Strabismus (AAPO&S)
    P.O. Box 193832 San Francisco, CA 94119
    Tel (415) 561-8505
    *This is the professional association for pediatric
    ophthalmologists in the US and around the
    world.*

2. The AAPO&S Home Page
    http://medaapos.bu.edu
    *This is the best single source of information
    about a wide range of pediatric ophthalmology
    concerns, including a question and answer
    service. It can direct people with enquiries to
    specific sources of information.*

3. Library of Congress, Division of the
    Blind and Physically Handicapped
    1291 Taylor Street N.W.
    Washington, DC 20213
    Tel (202) 376-6289
    *Offers a bibliography of readings for parents
    of handicapped children.*

4. Blind Children's Fund
    2875 NorthwindDrive, Suite 211
    East Lansing, MI 44823-5040
    Tel (517) 333-1725
    *Provides information for parents of preschool
    children with severe visual handicaps.*

5. The Lighthouse National Center for Vision and
    Child Development
    111 East 59th Street
    New York, NY 10022
    Tel (800) 334-5497 or (212)821-9200
    *Vision rehabilitation organization providing
    low vision services, education, research and
    advocacy.*

6. Pediatric Projects Inc.
    P.O. Box 1880
    Santa Monica, CA 90406
    *Provides a bibliography of books for children on
    vision and vision impairments*

7. American Printing House for the Blind
    1839 Frankfort Avenue
    P.O. Box 6085
    Louisville, KY 402060085
    Tel (502) 8952405

8. American Foundation for the Blind
    15 West 16th Street
    New York, NY 10011
    Tel (800) 232-5463 or (212)620-2043

9. The Institute for Families of Blind Children
    P.O. Box 54700, Mailstop #111
    Los Angeles, CA 90054-0700
    Tel (213) 6694649

10. National Association for Parents of the
    Visually Impaired
    P.O. Box 317
    Watertown, MA 02272-0317
    Tel (800) 562-6265 or (617) 972-7441

11. National Children's Eye Care Foundation
    P.O. Box 795069
    Dallas, TX 75379-5069
    Tel (972) 407-0404

12. Helen Keller Services for the Blind
    57 Willoughby Street
    Brooklyn, NY 11201
    Tel (718) 522-2122

13. The Center for the Partially Sighted
    720 Wilshire Boulevard, Suite 200
    Santa Monica, CA 90401-1713

14. Sturge-Weber Foundation
    8135 Run Drive, S.E.
    Olympia, WA 98503

15. National Organization for Albinism
    and Hypopigmentation (NOAH)
    1530 Locust Street #29
    Philadelphia, PA 19102
    Tel (800) 473-2310 or (215) 545-2322

16. National Marfan Foundation
    382 Main Street
    Port Washington, NY 10050

17. National Nerurofibromatosis Foundation
    95 Pine Street, 16th Floor
    New York, NY 10005

21 Dyslexia: Why Johnny Can't Read

with Frank R. Vellutino, Ph.D.*

*J*ohnny Lawlor was the perfect all-round kid. He was friendly, warm and outgoing — popular with his friends and even comfortable around their parents. He was an engaging conversationalist, clearly a bright child. But he wasn't doing well in second grade.

Johnny's problem was that he couldn't read as well as his classmates. When he tried to read, he just couldn't sound out or understand the words. He would lose his place and skip lines. He would complain that his eyes were tired, and he'd get a headache. As the school year wore on, the other kids made more progress and Johnny fell further behind. He became increasingly frustrated, embarrassed and discouraged.

Johnny's teacher called his mother in for a conference, and she confirmed what Mrs. Lawlor had suspected: Johnny had a severe reading problem. The teacher called it dyslexia.

Reading is the foundation of learning in our culture, essential to success in school and in many careers. Dyslexia means, simply, difficulty with reading. A variety of other names have been used since the problem was first described a century ago. A synonym currently in vogue is reading disability.

Dyslexia has been a confusing entity for parents, teachers, and even eye doctors. Because the cause remains somewhat obscure and because reading is so important, it has become a focus of controversy. Children and their parents have been subjected to a wide variety of "quick fix" treatments, for which there is little scientific basis or empiric evidence of success.

The precise incidence of dyslexia obviously depends on where we draw the line between normal and poor readers. At any grade level, and even among adults, reading proficiency falls in a normal, "bell-

* Professor of Psychology, Director of Child Research and Study Center, University at Albany, State University of New York.

shaped" distribution. Most people read at about an average level, a few are much better, and a few are much worse. Using different definitions, various studies have concluded that between 5% and 20% of Americans are dyslexic.

The problem typically becomes apparent in elementary school, and it usually involves spelling and writing, as well as reading. In the past, boys were thought to have the problem much more commonly than girls. Recent evidence, however, attributes some of this difference to a school referral bias. Boys tend to be less attentive and more disruptive in the classroom and may be more likely labeled dyslexic as a result.

What Causes Dyslexia?

Some dyslexics are limited by their intelligence. Some come from socially disadvantaged environments where reading readiness skills are not developed during the preschool years. Some children can't learn to read because they can't see the words or hear the teacher's instructions. Others may have trouble because they are hypoglycemic or because they have an occult seizure disorder.

Johnny's reading disability is primary, not secondary to some other problem with his eyes, ears, general health, or social circumstances. His case is typical. Despite normal intelligence, social background and overall health, he has fallen further and further behind his peers in elementary school. The preponderance of informed opinion attributes his problem to an isolated defect in processing written language. Most dyslexic children can be treated with educational remediation. Many have found ingenious ways to compensate and have had extremely successful careers. Discount broker Charles Schwab studied from his roommate's college notebook and often got better grades than the roommate. Vice President Nelson Rockefeller had his secretaries type a few key words that he used in giving his speeches. Some successful dyslexics even think they are better able to use intuitive reasoning as a result of their reading disability. Thomas Edison reportedly is one good example.

The defect itself may be genetically determined. Dyslexia certainly occurs more frequently in children who have close relatives who are poor readers, and recent research has implicated a specific gene on the 6th chromosome. Ultrastructural and electrophysiologic studies have identified subtle changes in the language areas of dyslexics' brains.

How we learn to read

To better understand why Johnny can't read, let's first explore how we normally learn reading skills. Reading depends on our ability t recognize words and their component sounds (called phonemes). We must orient and sequence letters and words, invest them with meaning, and store them in our memory for later retrieval. There are two basic strategies for recognizing phonemes.

The first, called phonetic decoding, relies on recognition of letter sounds and makes use of families of words (nut/cut/hut; raid/maid/paid). But some English words are difficult to "sound out" and have different meanings—and even pronunciations—depending on their context. For example, put and said don't belong in the above families, though they appear to. And bough and rough, already phonetic exceptions, are pronounced differently from each other.

The second decoding strategy, called whole-word recognition, takes advantage of context to identify words that are difficult to sound out. But whole-word recognition can be difficult when words are visually similar. Consider, for example, was and saw, or pot and top, which can be easily reversed.

Clearly, excessive reliance on either strategy can be responsible for poor reading performance. The best readers are facile with both, and the worst are unable to use either.

The eyes and reading

During reading the eyes "jump" in small steps, called *saccades*, across the page from left to right. A few right-to-left saccades also occur. Words, or groups of words, are perceived during the brief periods of fixation, between one-twentieth and one-half second in length, between saccades. Vision is effectively suppressed during saccades; otherwise we would be aware of the print moving past us as we move our eyes. (Larger saccades are generated by faster readers, especially with easier text.)

Eye movements of dyslexics are characterized by shorter saccades, more right-to-left saccades, and more fixation time between saccades. These differences result from the difficulty dyslexics experience decoding. They spend more time between saccades because they are struggling to make sense of the words they see. They make shorter saccades because they are unable to decode long segments of text. And they "back up" frequently to recheck the words they have already been over so they can get meaning from them. A normal reader might exhibit a similar eye movement pattern if presented a complicated and unfamiliar technical document.

Children who have even the most severe disturbance of their eye movements, for example congenital fibrosis or Moebius syndrome, can read normally, since less than 5 degrees of eye movement is needed for most lines of text. Indeed, the incidence of a wide range of eye disorders is similar among normal and dyslexic elementary students. It is exceptionally rare that ophthalmologic treatment — of strabismus, amblyopia, accommodative or convergence insufficiency, or even refractive error —is adequate or even appropriate intervention for children who present solely because of reading disability.

In the past, "mirror reading" or reversal errors, which are common among dyslexics, were thought to reflect an innate tendency for the eye to "see" print backwards. We now understand that such errors merely reflect excessive reliance on whole-word decoding. Dyslexics do not exhibit such reversals with other than written letters, and can reproduce words from an unfamiliar alphabet as well as can normal readers.

Treatments that don't work

Despite the absence of convincing scientific evidence to support them, a variety of "quick fix" treatments have found a receptive audience among desperate parents.

"Vision training" or "vision therapy" may be the most commonly advocated. Based on the assumption that visual impairments are responsible for difficulty orienting or sequencing letters or words, such programs include eye exercises to alleviate strabismus, amblyopia, disorders of accommodation, and faulty eye movements. Children are typically prescribed bifocals, may be given diets or megavitamins, and are supervised in "eye tracking" or similar exercises for prolonged periods.

Evidence for the purported visual defects is unconvincing, and no appropriately controlled study has demonstrated benefit from vision training. As a result, almost all medical doctors reject such programs. Indeed, the American Academy of Pediatrics, the American Academy of Ophthalmology, and the American Association for Pediatric Ophthalmology and Strabismus have all issued statements that vision training is ineffective.

Other treatments recommended for dyslexia include "motor therapy," which includes jumping on trampolines and walking on balance beams in order to stimulate word recognition. "Sequential processing therapy" involves the ordering of pictures or toys in an effort to sensitize the child to order letters and words. A variety of colored lenses have been prescribed on the unproven assumption that dyslexics' retinas are sensitive to light of different wavelengths. Other treatments have been directed at alleviating an unspecified inner ear defect. None of these treatments has been demonstrated to be effective in a properly controlled study.

What parents and primary care physicians can do

A more appropriate approach is to investigate each child's specific problem so that alternate strategies to facilitate word decoding might be developed. Usually such testing is done through the school system, supervised by an educational psychologist. Sometimes an outside evaluation is warranted. Parents should be aware of their right to receive remedial education treatment necessary for their child to succeed in school to his or her full potential. Perhaps a change in teacher or class level is appropriate, or the involvement of a reading teacher or a tutor. Whatever the intervention, it is best started early, before the child becomes so discouraged that his or her self image is permanently damaged. Parents can help by reading with their child daily and providing support.

Pediatricians and family physicians are often consulted, either by the parents or the school system. It is important to check the child's hearing, vision and neurologic status to be certain that treatable medical conditions are not overlooked. If a concern is evident in this regard, referral to the appropriate specialist for consultation can be considered. Pediatric ophthalmologists often see patients like Johnny after they have found their way into vision therapy programs and the parents seek another opinion. The role of the ophthalmologist is to be certain that there is no organic visual system pathology and to guide the family in the direction of effective educational remediation.

The primary care physician can be most helpful in supporting this approach and in cautioning the family against "quick fix" solutions. All involved must avoid conveying the impression that "nothing's wrong." On the contrary, something very serious may be wrong, but it is unlikely to have a medical or visual basis. It should be investigated and treated in an educational setting. The prognosis is actually very favorable. If appropriate remedial education is started by the second grade, 85% of dyslexic children will catch up to grade level within two years.

If appropriate remedial education is started by the second grade, 85% of dyslexic children will catch up to grade level within two years.

≈ঽ

After the conference at school, Johnny was evaluated with a variety of tests that took two days to finish. Afterward, he began to work with a reading teacher several hours a week and with a tutor on Saturday mornings. Though progress was slow, reading was getting to be less painful. He was no longer embarrassed when the teacher called on him to read aloud.

Glossary

A

abducens (ab-DU-senz). Sixth cranial nerve. Motor nerve that innervates the lateral rectus muscle, enabling each eye to rotate outward (away from nose). Originates in lower pons area of the brainstem; enters the orbit through the superior orbital fissure.

abducens palsy, lateral rectus *(or)* **6th nerve palsy**. Partial or total loss of function of the 6th (abducens) cranial nerve. The affected eye deviates inward (esotropia) and has defective ability to turn out beyond the midline (abduct) since it no longer receives adequate innervation; thus the deviation becomes greater and more apparent when both eyes rotate toward the affected side.

abrasion, corneal abrasion. Scraped area of corneal surface accompanied by loss of superficial tissue (epithelium).

AC/A ratio (accommodative convergence/accommodation ratio). Numerical expression for the relationship between the amount both eyes simultaneously turn inward (converge) and the amount their lenses increase in power (accommodate). In normal individuals this ratio averages 5:1. Accommodative convergence is expressed in prism diopters (Δ); accommodation is expressed in diopters (D).

accommodation (uh-kah-muh-DAY-shun). Increase in optical power by the eye in order to maintain a clear image (focus) as objects are moved closer. Occurs through a process of ciliary muscle contraction and zonular relaxation that causes the elastic-like lens to "round up" and increase its optical power.

accommodative convergence. See CONVERGENCE.

accommodative convergence/accommodation ratio. See AC/A RATIO.

accommodative effort syndrome. Eyestrain and blurred vision at near that results from excessive focusing effort of the eye's crystalline lens, to see near objects clearly.

accommodative esotropia (ee-soh-TROH-pee-uh). See ESOTROPIA.

achromatopsia (ay-kroh-muh-TAHP-see-uh), **monochromacy**. Rare inability to distinguish colors. Nonprogressive; hereditary.

acuity. See VISUAL ACUITY.

add. 1. Amount of plus power required for near use (over eyeglass correction for distance). 2. Plus lens fused to corrective eyeglasses (usually lower part); used for near work to compensate for the decrease in focusing ability (accommodation) that occurs normally with age.

adhesive syndrome. See CICATRICIAL STRABISMUS.

Adie's pupil (AY-deez), **pupillotonia, tonic pupil**. Disorder characterized by slow pupillary constriction to light, with sluggish redilation and decreased focusing ability for near (accommodation). Unilateral; at first the affected pupil is larger, later smaller than in the fellow eye. Seen with diseases of, or injury to, the ciliary ganglion, often in young women.

adjustable sutures. Surgical stitches that can be shortened or lengthened after surgery to obtain better eye alignment. May be used in reattaching an extraocular muscle.

afferent pupillary defect (AF-ur-unt). See MARCUS-GUNN PUPIL.

after-cataract. See SECONDARY CATARACT.

albinism (ocular). See OCULAR ALBINISM.

allergic conjunctivitis. See CONJUNCTIVITIS.

alternate cover test (ACT). See COVER TEST.

alternate prism + cover test (APCT). See COVER TEST.

alternate day esotropia (ee-suh-TROH-pee-uh). See ESOTROPIA.

alternating esotropia (ee-suh-TROH-pee-uh). See ESOTROPIA.

alternating strabismus (struh-BIZ-mus). See STRABISMUS.

alternating sursumduction, double *(or)* **dissociated double hypertropia, dissociated vertical deviation**. Eye deviation in which one eye floats upward and rolls outward (extorsion) whenever the two eyes are not working together, e.g., when one eye is covered.

amblyopia (am-blee-OH-pee-uh), "**lazy eye**." Decreased vision in one or both eyes without detectable anatomic damage in the eye or visual pathways. Usually uncorrectable by optical means (e.g., eyeglasses).

    ametropic: (am-uh-TROH-pik): amblyopic eye that has a high uncorrected refractive error (usually hyperopia or astigmatism). Vision may improve after several months of eyeglass correction.

    anisometropic: (an-ni-suh-muh-TROH-pik): decreased vision in the eye with the greater optical error; occurs when the eyes have significant difference in refraction. Vision may improve after several months of eyeglass correction.

    deprivation: follows central fixation disuse (due to cloudy cornea, cataract, droopy lid, etc.).

    a. ex anopsia: same as DISUSE (below). Term becoming obsolete.

    occlusion: 1. Caused by prolonged patching of the better-seeing eye to promote use of the weaker eye; usually reversible. 2. Same as DEPRIVATION (above).

    a. of disuse: amblyopic eye that has lost form discrimination after central fixation disuse (due to cloudy cornea, cataract, droopy lid, etc.).

    refractive: associated with large uncorrected refractive error (ametropia) or difference in refraction between the two eyes (anisometropia). Vision may improve after several months of eyeglass correction.

    strabismic: associated with a continuous eye deviation (usually inward) that begins before a child's visual acuity stabilizes. Can usually be reversed during the first 9 years of life by occlusion of the non-affected eye (often for months).

ametropia (am-uh-TROH-pee-uh). Any optical error (e.g. myopia) that can be corrected by eyeglasses or contact lenses.

amplitudes, fusional amplitudes. See VERGESNCE ABILITY.

angle. See ANTERIOR CHAMBER ANGLE.

anisocoria (an-i-suh-KOR-ee-uh). Unequal pupil size (difference of 1 mm or more).

anomalous (or) **abnormal retinal correspondence (ARC)**. Binocular sensory adaptation to compensate for a long-standing eye deviation; fovea of the straight (non-deviated) eye and a non-foveal retinal point of the deviated eye work together, sometimes permitting single binocular vision despite the misalignment.

anophthalmia (an-ahf-THAL-mee-uh), **anophthalmos**. Absence of the eyeball.

anterior chamber (AC). Fluid-filled space inside the eye between the iris and the innermost corneal surface (endothelium).

anterior chamber angle, angle. Junction of the front surface of the iris and back surface of the cornea, where aqueous fluid filters out of the eye. Incorporates nearby structures, which include Schlemm's canal, scleral spur, trabecular meshwork, Schwalbe's line, and iris processes.

anterior chamber cleavage syndrome, mesodermal dysgenesis of cornea, Peter anomaly. Central cornea malformation characterized by adherence of the iris to Descemet's membrane and the endothelium (innermost corneal layer). May be associated with iridocorneal angle abnormalities and cataract.

anterior segment. Front third of the eyeball; includes structures located between the front surface of the cornea and the vitreous.

anterior synechia (sin-EE-kee-uh). Adhesions binding the front of the iris to the innermost corneal surface.

anterior uveitis (yu-vee-l-tis), **iridocyclitis**. Inflammation of iris, anterior chamber or ciliary body. Causes pain, tearing, blurred vision, constricted pupil and a red (congested) eye.

anterior vitrectomy. Removal of front portion of vitreous tissue. Used for preventing or treating vitreous loss during cataract or corneal surgery, or to remove misplaced vitreous, as in aphakic pupillary block glaucoma.

A pattern. Horizontal eye misalignment in which an inward turning (esotropic) eye deviates more on up-gaze than on down-gaze, or an outward turning (exotropic) eye deviates more on down-gaze than up-gaze.

aphake (AY-fayk). Patient whose crystalline lens has been removed, e.g., after cataract extraction.

aphakia (ay-FAY-kee-uh). Absence of the eye's crystalline lens, e.g., after cataract extraction.

aphakic correction (ay-FAY-kik). Contact or eyeglass lens that replaces optical power lost after cataract extraction, or lens loss from any cause.

applanation tonometer (tuh-NAHM-ih-tur). Determines intraocular pressure by measuring the force required to flatten a small area of central cornea. Usually attaches to slit lamp. Examples: Draeger and Goldmann tonometers.

aqueous (AY-kwee-us), **aqueous humor**. Clear, watery fluid that fills the space between the back surface of the cornea and the front surface of the vitreous, bathing the lens. Produced by the ciliary processes. Nourishes the cornea, iris, and lens and maintains intraocular pressure.

aqueous flare, flare, Tyndall effect. Scattering of a slit lamp light beam when it is directed into the anterior chamber; occurs when aqueous has increased protein. Sign of iris or ciliary body inflammation (iritis).

asthenopia (as-then-OH-pee-uh). Vague eye discomfort arising from use of the eyes; may consist of eyestrain, headache, and/or browache. May be related to uncorrected refractive error or poor fusional amplitudes.

astigmatism (uh-STIG-muh-tiz-um). Optical defect in which refractive power is not uniform in all directions (meridians). Light rays entering the eye are bent unequally by different meridians, with maximum and minimum powers 90° to one another, which prevents formation of a sharp point focus on the retina. Instead, light rays form two focal lines separated by a focal zone. Usually results from corneal asphericity. Corrected by a cylindrical (toric) eyeglass or contact lens.

B

band keratopathy (kehr-uh-TAHP-uh-thee). Horizontal band of calcium deposits in superficial layers of the cornea; associated with chronic uveitis and other chronic ocular diseases.

Barkan's membrane. Thin membrane covering trabeculum. May have etiologic significance in congenital glaucoma.

base-down prism (BD). A prism whose thickest edge is downward; when placed in front of an eye, it moves the image upward and thus can be used to measure or treat an upward eye deviation (hypertropia, hyperphoria). Sometimes incorporated into eyeglasses.

base-in prism (BI). A prism whose thickest edge is inward (toward the nose); when placed in front of an eye, it moves the image outward and thus can be used to measure or treat an outward eye deviation (exotropia, exophoria). Sometimes incorporated into eyeglasses.

base-out prism (BO). A prism whose thickest edge is outward (toward the ear); when placed in front of an eye, it moves the image inward and thus can be used to measure or treat an inward eye deviation (esotropia, esophoria). Sometimes incorporated into eyeglasses.

base-up prism (BU). A prism whose thickest edge is upward. When placed in front of an eye, it moves the image downward and thus can be used to measure or treat downward eye deviations (hypotropia, hypophoria). Sometimes incorporated into eyeglasses.

Bell's palsy, facial palsy. Paralysis of muscles innervated by the 7th (facial) cranial nerve, which move facial structures surrounding the brow, eyelids and mouth. Eyelid on the affected side does not close properly, so corneal drying may become a problem.

Bell's phenomenon. Upward and outward deviation of the eyes during sleep or with forcible closure of the eyelids.

Bielschowsky head tilt test (beel-SHAH/OW-skee). The head is tilted to one shoulder, then the other, to distinguish between a truly weak vertical muscle in one eye and an apparently weak vertical muscle in the other eye.

binocular depth perception, stereopsis, stereoscopic vision, 3rd grade fusion. Visual blending of two similar images (one falling on each retina) into one, with visual perception of solidity and depth.

binocular fixation pattern (BFP). Used in conjunction with a cover test to determine whether one eye is more often straight and preferred for fixation than the other.

binocularity. Ability to use both eyes together.

blepharoconjunctivitis (BLEF-uh-roh-kun-junk-tuh-VI-tis). Inflammation of the conjunctiva (membrane covering white of eye, undersurface of lids, and margins of upper and lower eyelids).

blepharoptosis (blef-uh-rahp-TOH-sis). See PTOSIS.

blindness. Inability to see.

> **cerebral**: same as CORTICAL (below).

> **cortical**: caused by damage to the blood supply of the visual areas in the brain's occipital cortices. Retina appears normal; visually-evoked electrical response (VER) is markedly diminished.

> **legal**: best-corrected visual acuity of 20/200 or less, or reduction in visual field to 20° or less, in the better-seeing eye.

> **night**: see NIGHT BLINDNESS.

blocked tear duct, nasolacrimal duct obstruction. Incomplete opening of a tear duct; causes continuous tearing.

"blown pupil," fixed dilated pupil. Enlarged pupil that does not constrict in response to a light stimulus, a near object, or a light stimulus in the other eye.

blowout fracture. Break in the bony orbital floor or walls caused by blunt trauma to eye or orbit. Intraorbital contents are pushed into one or more of the paranasal sinuses.

botulinum toxin (bah-tchu-LI-num). Poison derived from botulinum bacterium. Paralyzes muscle fibers temporarily. Used as an alternative or addition to surgery to correct eye misalignments or to paralyze a facial nerve causing uncontrollable lid spasms. Trade names: Botox, Oculinum.

Brown's syndrome. See SUPERIOR OBLIQUE TENDON SHEATH SYNDROME.

Brushfield spots. Gray or brown spots on the iris, associated with mongolism (Down's syndrome). Also found in many normal children.

buphthalmos (boof-THAL-mus), **hydrophthalmos**. Abnormally large eyeball ("ox-eye") caused by glaucoma in a young, stretchable eye.

C

calipers. Measuring device with two adjustable arms, for determining thickness, diameter, or distance between two points.

canaliculus (kan-uh-LIK-yu-lus), **lacrimal canaliculus**. Tiny channel in each eyelid that forms part of the tear drainage system. Begins at the lacrimal punctum in both upper and lower lids, joining to form the common canaliculus, which leads to the tear (lacrimal) sac and then through the nasolacrimal duct into the nose. Plural: canaliculi. .

> **common c**: tiny channel under the skin (between the eyelids and the nose) formed by the junction of the upper and lower canaliculi; leads to the lacrimal sac.

capsule, lens capsule. Elastic bag enveloping the eye's crystalline lens. Helps control the shape of the lens for accommodation.

> **anterior capsule**: front of the capsule; lies in the posterior chamber just behind the iris.

> **posterior capsule**: rear of the capsule; lies against the anterior hyaloid membrane of the vitreous.

cardinal positions of gaze. Six positions (right, left, up + right, down + right, up + left, down + left) used for testing the six pairs of muscles involved in eye movement coordination.

cataract. Opacity or cloudiness of the crystalline lens, which may prevent a clear image from forming on the retina. Surgical removal of lens may be necessary if visual loss becomes significant, with lost optical power replaced with an intraocular lens, contact lens or aphakic spectacles. May be congenital or caused by trauma, disease, or age.

cataract extraction. Removal of a cloudy lens from the eye.

> **extracapsular**: method that leaves the rear lens capsule intact.

> **intracapsular**: complete removal of lens with its capsule, usually by cryoextraction.

cat eye syndrome. Chromosome abnormality characterized by developmental and mental retardation, ear tags, macula underdevelopment, optic nerve degeneration, and an incomplete iris that looks like a cat's eye.

cat's eye pupil. Unusual whitish glint in the normally black pupil; resembles the reflection seen when a light shines into a cat's eye at night.

"cells and flare." Accumulation of white blood cells and increased protein in the aqueous, visible on slit-lamp examination of the anterior chamber. Associated with inflammation of the iris and/or ciliary body.

cellulitis (sel-yu-LI-tis). Infection or inflammation of tissues.

> **orbital**: infection of orbital contents, often caused by streptococci or staphylococci. Produces swelling and redness of lids, bulging eye (proptosis), limitation of eye movement, and swelling of orbital tissues. Usually spreads from infected ethmoid, spheroid, maxillary or frontal sinuses.

> **pre-septal**: swelling or infection of eyelid tissue in front of the orbital septum. Does not affect the eyeball.

chalazion (kuh-LAY-zee-un). Inflamed lump in a meibomian gland (in the eyelid). Inflammation usually subsides, but may need surgical removal. Sometimes called an internal hordeolum. Plural: chalazia.

cherry-red spot. Apparent color change in the fovea (retinal area of sharpest vision). Results from opacification of the inner retinal layers around it, allowing red color of choroidal circulation to stand out. Occurs in central retinal artery occlusion and Tay-Sachs disease.

chiasm (KI-az-um), **optic chiasm**. X-shaped part of the retina-to-brain nerve chain, where retinal nerve fibers from the nasal side of both eyes cross to the opposite side and optic nerves from the two eyes join and form the optic tracts. Located at the base of the brain just above the pituitary gland.

choked disc. See PAPILLEDEMA.

choroid (KOR-oyd). Vascular (major blood vessel) layer of the eye lying between the retina and sclera. Provides nourishment to outer layers of the retina. Forms part of the uvea, along with the ciliary body and iris.

cicatricial strabismus (struh-BIZ-mus), **adhesive syndrome**. Limitation of eye movement with damage and scarring of the muscle cone or supportive tissue (e.g., Tenon's capsule and fat); found after orbital trauma or surgery.

ciliary body. Circumferential tissue inside the eye composed of the ciliary muscle (involved in lens accommodation and control of intraocular pressure) and 70 ciliary processes that produce aqueous.

ciliary flush, ciliary hyperemia (or) **injection**. External eye redness caused by congestion of blood vessels surrounding the corneo- scleral junction (limbus). Associated with corneal inflammation, iritis or acute angle closure glaucoma.

Cloquet's canal (kloh-KAYZ), **hyaloid canal**. Pathway within the vitreous that extends from the optic disc to the lens. In the fetus, contains the hyaloid artery, which disappears before birth, though the canal remains.

coloboma (kah-luh-BOH-muh). Cleft or defect in normal continuity of a part of the eye, e.g., absence of lower segment of optic nerve head, choroid, ciliary body, iris, lens or eyelid. Caused by improper fusion of fetal fissure during gestation. May be associated with other abnormalities, including a small eye (microphthalmia). Plural: colobomata.

color blindness. See ROD MONOCHROMACY.

comitant strabismus (KAH-muh-tunt struh-BIZ-mus), **concomitant strabismus**. See STRABISMUS.

common canaliculus (kan-uh-LIK-yu-luhs). See CANALICULUS.

cone degeneration, cone dystrophy. Degeneration of retinal receptors (primarily cones); results in progressive, marked decrease in vision and loss of color discrimination. Hereditary. No known treatment.

confrontation fields. Screening method for gross visual field defects, using the examiner's eye as a fixation point and his moving fingers as peripheral targets.

confusion. Simultaneous perception of two objects in the same location in space. Occurs at the onset of an eye deviation, when fovea of each eye is stimulated by a different object.

congenital amaurosis (am-uh-ROH-sis), **Leber's congenital amaurosis**. Blindness or near-blindness in both eyes; may be accompanied by nystagmus, sensitivity to light, and sunken eyes. Marked reduction in retinal function, seen on an electroretinogram.

congenital bulbar paralysis. See MÖBIUS' SYNDROME.

congenital esotropia (ee-soh-TROH-pee-uh). See ESOTROPIA.

congenital fibrosis syndrome. Inability of the eyes to look upward or to either side. Characterized by eyes fixed in downward direction, drooping eyelids (ptosis), and chin-up head position. Usually hereditary.

congenital glaucoma (glaw-KOH-muh). See GLAUCOMA.

congenital nystagmus (ni-stag-mus). See NYSTAGMUS.

congenital oculomotor apraxia (COMA) (ay-PRAK-see-uh), **Cogan's congenital oculomotor apraxia**. Inability to make voluntary eye movements; results in head-thrusting to bring the eyes into desired gaze positions. Usually improves with age.

congenital stationary night blindness (CSNB). Non-progressive retinal disorder characterized by poor night vision; rod function is abnormal. Retina appears normal. Hereditary.

conjugate movement (KAHN-juh-gut), **conjunctive** (or) **gaze movement, version**. Parallel movements of both eyes.

conjunctiva (kahn-junk-TI-vuh). Transparent mucous membrane covering the outer surface of the eyeball except the cornea, and lining the inner surfaces of the eyelids. Plural: conjunctivae.

    bulbar: portion that covers the external eyeball.

    palpebral: portion that lines the eyelids.

conjunctival hyperemia (hi-pur-EE-mee-uh). See CONJUNCTIVAL INJECTION.

conjunctival injection, conjunctival hyperemia. Eye redness caused by congestion of blood vessels in the conjunctiva (membrane covering white of eye and inner eyelids); most prominent near the fornix and decreasing toward the corneo-scleral junction (limbus). Associated with all types of conjunctivitis.

conjunctival sac. See CUL-DE-SAC.

conjunctivitis (kun-junk-tih-VI-tis), "**pink eye**." Inflammation of the conjunctiva (mucus membrane that covers white of eye and inner eyelid surfaces). Characterized by discharge, grittiness, redness and swelling. Usually viral in origin; may be contagious.

    acute: having sudden onset.

    allergic: hypersensitivity to foreign substances. Characterized by discharge, itching, irritation, swelling, tearing, redness, and light sensitivity. The discharge contains a large number of white blood cells (eosinophils).

    atopic: allergic reaction to pollens; usually accompanies hay fever.

    bacterial: caused by infection; characterized by muco-pus discharge, redness, and a gritty feeling.

    chronic: persistent or intermittent.

    contact: caused by allergy or by irritation from eye medications or cosmetics used near the eye.

    dermato- involves bulbar and palpebral conjunctiva as well as the skin near the eyelid margins.

    follicular: characterized by hundreds of tiny, glistening, translucent elevations (follicles) composed of Iymphoid tissue on undersurfaces of lids.

    Parinaud's oculo-glandular: characterized by conjunctival lesions surrounded by follicles, with fever and malaise. Rare; usually affects only one eye.

    vernal: allergic reaction (itching, mucous); numerous small lumps (papillae) form on palpebral conjunctiva. Affects children; recurs in warm summer months.

    viral: caused by a virus; characterized by discharge, grittiness, redness and swelling. Usually contagious.

consecutive esotropia (ee-suh-TROH-pee-uh). See ESOTROPOIA.

consecutive exotropia (eks-uh-TROH-pee-uh). See EXOTROPIA.

contact lens. See RIGID GAS PERMEABLE LENS, SILICONE LENS, SOFT LENS.

contralateral. Refers to the opposite eye or the opposite side of the body.

contralateral antagonist. Extraocular muscle whose action is opposite to that of another muscle in the opposite eye (e.g., right superior oblique, left superior rectus).

converge. 1. Refers to the coming together of light rays toward a focus. 2. To move both eyes inward (toward each other), usually in an effort to maintain single binocular vision as an object approaches.

convergence. Inward movement of both eyes toward each other, usually in an effort to maintain single binocular vision as an object approaches.

accommodative: portion of the range of inward rotation that occurs in response to an increase in optical power for focusing (accommodation) by the eyes' lenses.

fusional: amount the eyes can converge while maintaining single vision. Measured with graduated base-out prisms.

proximal: portion of convergence brought about by awareness of an object's nearness.

relative: amount of prism power that can be overcome while single clear binocular vision is maintained. May be positive or negative, depending on direction of the prism.

tonic: portion of convergence that results from changing from sleeping to the awake state.

voluntary: amount the eyes can voluntarily converge without regard to clarity or single image.

convergence amplitudes. Amount the eyes can turn inward before double vision occurs. Measured in prism diopters.

convergence insufficiency. Eye muscle problem in which the eyes cannot be pulled sufficiently inward (toward each other) to maintain single vision when attempting to fixate on a near object. Characterized by eye fatigue or double vision.

convergence spasm. Inward eye deviation (esotropia), usually accompanied by small pupils and by excessive accommodation (focusing power) that causes blurred distance vision (near vision remains clear). Usually related to an emotional problem or hysteria.

corectopia (kor-ek-TOH-pee-uh). Displacement of the pupil from its normal position.

cornea (KOR-nee-uh). Transparent front part of the eye that covers the iris, pupil and anterior chamber and provides most of an eye's optical power. Five layers: epithelium, Bowman's membrane, stroma, Decemet's membrane and endothelium.

corneal abrasion (KOR-nee-ul). Scraped area of corneal surface, accompanied by loss of superficial tissue (epithelium).

corneal transplant, corneal graft, keratoplasty. Replacement of a scarred or diseased cornea with clear corneal tissue from a donor.

corneal ulcer. Area of epithelial tissue loss from the corneal surface. Associated with inflammatory cells in the cornea and anterior chamber. May be caused by bacterial, fungal, or viral infection.

cover test (CT). Detects eye misalignment (tropia) or tendency toward misalignment (phoria).

alternate cover test: same as cross cover test (below).

alternate prism + cover test (APCT): as target is viewed, a prism is placed over one eye and a cover over the other eye; the cover is moved from eye to eye. Eye movement is noted as prism power is changed; power used when movement stops is the deviation measurement.

cross cover test: target is viewed while a cover is moved from eye to eye and the direction of each eye's movement is noted.

prism + alternate cover test: same as alternate prism + cover test (above).

cover/uncover test: as the subject views a fixation target, one eye is covered and other eye is observed for movement; then the cover is removed and movement of both eyes is noted.

simultaneous prism and cover test (SPCT): quantifies the constant component of an eye deviation (tropia). A prism held in front of a deviating eye eliminates any refixation movement as the straight, fixating eye is simultaneously covered.

craniofacial dysostosis (kray-nee-oh-FAY-shul dis-ahs-TOH-sis), **Crouzon's syndrome**. Characterized by multiple abnormalities of skull and jaw, e.g., short head, broad hooked nose, high palate, large earlobes, widely separated eyes, shallow orbits, optic nerve damage, corneal exposure, nystagmus, and outward eye deviation (exotropia).

cross cover test. See COVER TEST.

cross-eyes. See ESOTROPIA.

cross-fixation. Viewing an object in left gaze with the right eye, and an object in right gaze with the left eye. Frequently associated with a large infantile esotropia.

cul-de-sac, conjunctival sac, fornix. Loose pocket of conjunctiva between upper eyelid and eyeball or lower eyelid and eyeball; permits the eyeball to rotate freely.

cupped disc, cupping. Abnormal enlargement of the optic cup (depression in center of optic disc). Most commonly due to prolonged increase in intraocular pressure.

cyclitic membrane (si-KLIH-tik). Membrane of fibrous tissue and inflammatory cells that grows across the front surface of the vitreous. Can cause decrease in vision or even massive shrinkage (phthisis) of the eye. Results from extensive intraocular inflammations.

cycloplegia (si-kloh-PLEE-juh). Paralysis of the ciliary muscle, eliminating accommodation. Clinically accomplished with eyedrops that temporarily block the action of the parasympathetic nerves in the eye.

cycloversion (si-kloh-VUR-zhun). Tilting of vertical axes of both eyes in the same (right or left) direction.

D

dacryocystitis (DAK-ree-oh-sis-TI-tis). Inflammation of the tear sac. Associated with faulty tear drainage.

dacryocystorhinostomy (DCR) (DAK-ree-oh-sis-toh-ri-NAHS-toh-mee). Construction of a new tear drainage channel from the lacrimal sac into the nose.

dacryostenosis (dak-ree-oh-sten-OH-sis). Abnormally narrow opening of the tear sac.

depth perception. Awareness of the relative spatial location of objects, some being closer to the observer than others. See also BINOCULAR DEPTH PERCEPTION.

dermoid, dermoid cyst, epibulbar dermoid. Tumor containing skin elements such as epithelium, fat, and hair; usually found at the corneo-scleral junction (limbus) or the lateral side of the upper eyelid.

deviation. See STRABISMUS.

diopter (D) (di-AHP-tur). Unit to designate the refractive power of a lens, or the degree of light convergence or divergence. Equal to the reciprocal of a lens' focal length (in meters), e.g., a 2-diopter lens brings parallel rays of light to a focus at 1/2 m.

diplopia fields. 1. Determination of the amount and direction of double vision in each of the nine diagnostic eye positions, evaluated with a fixation light, red filter or Maddox rod and prisms. 2. Visual field analysis of both eyes simultaneously to distinguish areas of single vision from double vision.

disc. See OPTIC DISC.

disinsertion (dis-in-SUR-shun). Cutting an extraocular muscle free from its attachment on the eyeball. Used as a muscle weakening procedure to correct an eye deviation.

disjunctive vergence, disconjugate *(or)* **disjigate movement, vergence**. Movement of both eyes in opposite directions (toward or away from each other, up and down) to obtain or maintain single binocular vision.

dislocated lens. Partial or complete displacement of the crystalline lens from its normal position; caused by broken or absent zonules.

dissociated double hypertropia, dissociated vertical deviation. See ALTERNATING SURSUMDUCTION.

divergence. 1. Refers to the spreading apart of light rays as they leave an object or a minus-powered lens. 2.Outward (away from each other) eye rotation, usually in an effort to maintain single binocular vision.

    relative: amount of base-in prism that can be overcome while maintaining clear binocular single vision. Also called relative fusional divergence.

double hypertropia. See ALTERNATING SURSUMDUCTION.

double elevator palsy. Paralysis of extraocular muscles responsible for moving the eye upward (superior rectus, inferior oblique). May be associated with convergence, pupil and eyelid abnormalities.

Duane's syndrome, Duane's co-contraction *(or)* **retraction syndrome, Stilling-Turk-Duane retraction syndrome**. Eye muscle abnormality characterized by inability to move one eye outward past the midline and retraction of that eye into the orbit, with narrowing of the eyelid fissure on attempted movement of that eye toward the nose. Often accompanied by an inward eye deviation (esotropia).

duction (DUK-shun). Movement of one eye; refers to movement ability measured independently from that of the other eye.

dyslexia (dis-LEK-see-uh). Reading disability associated with problems in interpreting written symbols. Not related to visual acuity or intelligence, which are usually normal.

E

ectopia lentis. Partial displacement of the crystalline lens, caused by broken or absent zonules. May be hereditary.

ectropion (ek-TROH-pee-un). Outward turning of the upper or lower eyelid so that the lid margin does not rest against the eyeball, but falls or is pulled away. Can create corneal exposure with excessive drying, tearing, and irritation. Usually from aging.

electroretinogram (ERG) (eh-LEK-troh-RET-in-oh-gram). Electrophysiological measure of retinal function after light stimulation of retina. Consists of several wave forms, e.g., a-waves, which show rod and cone activity, and b-waves, which stem from Mueller and bipolar cells.

emmetropia (em-uh-TROH-pee-uh). Refractive state of having no refractive error when accommodation is at rest. Images of distant objects are focused sharply on the retina without the need for either accommodation or corrective lenses.

entropion (en-TROH-pee-un). Inward turning of upper or lower eyelid so that the lid margin rests against and rubs the eyeball.

enucleation (ee-nu-klee-AY-shun). Removal of the eyeball, leaving eye muscles and remaining orbital contents intact.

epiblepharon (ep-ee-BLEF-ur-ahn). Abnormal skin fold across the upper or lower eyelid.

epibulbar dermoid. See DERMOID.

epicanthal fold (ep-ee-KAN-thul), **epicanthus**. Vertical skin fold on either side of nose, hiding the caruncle. Present in all infants before bridge of nose is formed, and in most Oriental adults. May make normal eyes appear crossed.

epicanthus inversus (in-VUR-sus). Vertical skin fold arising from the lower eyelid and inserting laterally into the upper lid.

epidemic keratoconjunctivitis (EKC) (KEHR-uh-toh-kun-junk-tih-VI-tis). Contagious infection of the cornea and conjunctiva, caused by an adenovirus.

esophoria (E) (ee-soh-FOR-ee-uh). Tendency toward inward (toward nose) deviation of one eye when a cover is placed over that eye. When cover is removed, eye straightens. See also PHORIA.

esotropia (ET) (ee-soh-TROH-pee-uh), **convergent deviation, cross-eyes, internal strabismus**. Eye misalignment in which one eye deviates inward (toward nose) while the other fixates normally. Present even when both eyes are uncovered.

    accommodative: caused by overactive convergence response to the accommodative effort necessary to keep vision clear; more common in hyperopic children. Eyeglass correction for the hyperopia relaxes accommodation, allowing the eyes to remain properly aligned. Sometimes bifocals can correct the excessive inturning at near.

    acquired: appears after age 6 months; often helped by eyeglasses.

    alternate day: deviation follows a 48-hour cycle, alternating 24 hours of normal binocularity with 24 hours of one eye turning inward.

    alternating: deviation continuously changes between an inturningright eye and straight left eye, and an inturning left eye and straight right eye.

    A pattern: deviation greater in up- than in down-gaze.

    circadian heterotropia: same as ALTERNATE DAY (above).

    congenital: same as INFANTILE (below).

    consecutive: follows surgical correction of exotropia (outward deviation).

    cyclic strabismus: same as ALTERNATE DAY (above).

    infantile: found at birth or within first 6 months; usually a large deviation that requires surgery (unaffected by eyeglasses).

intermittent [E(T)]: occasional deviation; sometimes the eyes look straight ahead and work together normally, other times one eye deviates inward while the other fixates normally.

non-accommodative: excessive turning is not influenced by correcting the hyperopia (farsightedness).

sensory: follows loss of vision in the affected eye.

V pattern: deviation greater in down- than up-gaze.

excimer laser (EKS-ih-mur). Class of ultraviolet lasers (argon-fluoride type), wavelength 193 nm, used for photorefractive keratectomy (PRK). Excimer refers to the molecular reaction (photodisruption) that removes tissue without heating it or surrounding tissue. Combined with other technologies, e.g., automated lamellar keratoplasty (ALK) to produce LASIK (laser in situ keratomileusis).

excyclovergence. Outward rotation of both eyes (from 12 o'clock meridian) while maintaining single binocular vision.

exophoria (eks-uh-FOR-ee-uh). Tendency toward outward (away from nose) deviation of one eye when cover is placed over that eye. Eye straightens to align with uninvolved eye when cover is removed.

exophthalmos (eks-ahf-THAL-mus), **proptosis.** Abnormal protrusion or bulging forward of the eyeball.

exotropia (XT) (eks-oh-TROH-pee-uh), **divergent** (or) **external strabismus, wall-eyes.** Eye misalignment in which one eye deviates outward (away from nose) while the other fixates normally.

A pattern: deviation greater in down- than in up-gaze.

basic: measures the same at near (16 in.) as at distance (20 ft.).

consecutive: follows surgical correction of inward deviation (esotropia).

intermittent [X(T)]: sometimes eyes look straight ahead and work together; other times one eye deviates out while the other fixates normally.

secondary: gradually develops in an inturning eye.

sensory: follows loss of vision in the affected eye.

V pattern: deviation is greater in up- than in down-gaze.

extorsion, excycloduction. Outward rotation of one eye; the 12 o'clock meridian rolls away from the nose.

eye popping. 1. Self-inflicted finger pressure against upper and lower eyelid folds to push an eye partly out of its socket; may cause optic nerve compression. 2. An infant's spontaneously opening the lids in response to dimming the room lights; provides evidence of visual function.

eyestrain. See ASTHENOPIA.

F

facial palsy. See BELL'S PALSY.
Faden procedure. See RETROEQUATORIAL MYOPEXY.
farsightedness. See HYPEROPIA.
fascia bulbi. See TENON'S CAPSULE.
field of vision. See VISUAL FIELD.

fixate. To move an eye so that a viewed object is imaged on the fovea.

fixation. Coordinated accommodation and ocular movements that achieve and maintain the image of objects on the fovea.

fixation preference (FP). Use of a cover-uncover test to evaluate how well a misaligned eye maintains fixation.

flare. See AQUEOUS FLARE.

fluorescein (FLOR-uh-seen). Yellow-green dye that fluoresces when illuminated with light of specific wavelength, usually ultraviolet. Injected intravenously to study blood flow through the retina and choroid. Can also be applied directly to the cornea to detect abrasions or leakage from surgical wounds or to evaluate the fit of some contact lenses, or to the conjunctiva to evaluate tear drainage.

fluorescein angiography (FA) (an-jee-AHG-ruh-fee). Used for evaluating retinal, choroidal, and iris blood vessels, as well as any eye problems affecting them. Fluorescein dye is injected into an arm vein, then rapid, sequential photographs are taken of the eye as the dye circulates.

follicles. Tiny, glistening, translucent (lymphoid) elevations on the undersurface of eyelids. Associated with viral conjunctival inflammation.

force duction test (DUK-shun), **traction test.** Forcibly moving the eyeball into different positions by grasping the anesthetized conjunctiva and episclera with forceps at the corneo-scleral junction (limbus). For determining if there are any mechanical restrictions to movement.

forced generation test. For determining function of a paralyzed extraocular muscle; patient attempts to move anesthetized eye held with forceps.

forced preferential looking (FPL). Specific method of preferential looking technique. Vision evaluated in preverbal children by noting whether they choose blank side of a large rectangular card or the side with spatial frquency stripes.

fornix. See CUL-DE-SAC.

fourth nerve palsy, superior oblique palsy. Head tilt and upward eye deviation (hypertropia) caused by damage to the 4th (trochlear) cranial nerve; reduces the effectiveness of the superior oblique muscle.

fovea (FOH-vee-uh), **fovea centralis.** Central pit in macula that produces sharpest vision. Contains a high concentration of cones and no retinal blood vessels. Plural: foveae.

fusion. Perceptual blending of two similar images, one from each eye, into one image that is maintained as the eyes converge or diverge.

1st grade: the superimposed images are dissimilar.

2nd grade: vergence movements allow blending of the similar images into one as the images move off the fovea.

3rd grade: binocular perception of depth (stereopsis) as slightly dissimilar images are blended.

fusional amplitudes. See VERGENCE ABILITY.
fusional convergence. See CONVERGENCE.

G

gas permeable lens (GP). See RIGID GAS PERMEABLE LENS.
gaze palsy. Inability of the eyes to make parallel movements in a specific direction.

giant papillary conjunctivitis (GPC). Allergic type of conjunctival inflammation often associated with continuous wearing of contact lenses. Hard, flat papillae form a cobblestone pattern on undersurface of the upper eyelid.

glaucoma. Group of diseases characterized by increased intraocular pressure resulting in damage to the optic nerve and retinal nerve fibers. Documented by typical visual field defects and increased size of optic cup. A common cause of preventable vision loss. May be treated by prescription drugs or surgery.

> **absolute**: end-stage, in which pressure remains elevated and vision is completely lost.

> **angle closure**: sudden rise in intraocular pressure. Aqueous fluid behind the iris cannot pass through the pupil and pushes the iris forward, preventing aqueous drainage through the angle (pupillary block mechanism). Occurs in patients who have narrow anterior chamber angles.

> **chronic open angle**: same as OPEN ANGLE (below).

> **congenital**: high intraocular pressure accompanied by hazy corneas and large eyes (buphthalmos) in newborn, resulting from developmental abnormalities in the anterior chamber angle that obstruct the intraocular fluid drainage mechanism. Characteristic symptoms are tearing, light sensitivity (photophobia) and uncontrolled blinking (blepharospasm). Requires early surgical correction.

> **infantile**: same as CONGENITAL (above).

> **open angle**: most common type; gradual blockage of aqueous outflow from the eye despite an apparently open anterior chamber angle. If untreated, results in gradual, painless, irreversible loss of vision. Usually in both eyes.

> **primary open angle (POAG)**: same as OPEN ANGLE.

> **secondary**: results from a known cause, such as inflammation, degeneration, trauma or tumor growths within the eye.

glioma (glee-OH-muh). Tumor derived from neuroglial components.

> **optic nerve glioma**: slow-growing, non-malignant congenital tumor of the optic nerve or optic chiasm composed of glial supportive cells. Often presents with eye protrusion (proptosis), enlarged optic foramen and decreased vision. Often seen with neurofibromatosis.

gonioscopy (goh-nee-AHS-koh-pee). Examination of the anterior chamber angle through a contact lens, using a slit lamp or modified hand-held microscope.

goniotomy (goh-nee-AHT-uh-mee). Incision made in trabecular meshwork. Used for treating congenital glaucoma.

Graves' disease, endocrine (or) **Graves' exophthalmos** (or) **ophthalmopathy, thyroid eye disease, thyrotoxic** (or) **thyrotropic exophthalmos**. Eye signs that may occur with excessive thyroid-related hormone concentration. Includes eyelid retraction, eyelid lag on downward gaze, corneal drying, eye bulging (proptosis), fibrotic extraocular muscles, and optic nerve inflammation.

Gunn pupil. See MARCUS-GUNN PUPIL.

H

hamartoma (ham-ahr-TOH-muh). Non-cancerous tumor mass resulting from faulty embryonic development. Composed of cells normally found at that site. Example: cavernous hemangioma.

hand movement (HM). Patient's ability to see movement of a waving hand at a specified distance, usually 1 ft. or less. Used when vision loss is too profound for counting fingers.

hemangioma (hee-man-jee-OH-muh). Tumor comprised of blood vessels or vessel elements.

> **capillary**: composed of small dilated blood vessels. On the skin, it appears as small bright red spots.

> **cavernous**: deep purplish tumor composed of large vascular channels. Usually located in the eyelids or in the orbit above and behind the lids. Tends to regress somewhat with age.

hemianopsia (hem-ee-uh-NAHP-see-uh), **hemianopia**. Non-seeing area in the right or left half of the visual field.

heterophoria (het-ur-uh-FOR-ee-uh). See PHORIA.

heterotropia (het-ur-uh-TROH-pee-uh). See STRABISMUS.

Hirschberg test. Determines relative position of corneal light reflexes on both eyes, to allow estimation of a misaligned eye's deviation.

hordeolum (hor-DEE-oh-lum).

> **external (stye)**: pustular infection of the oil glands of Zeis, located in the eyelash follicles at eyelid margins.

> **internal**: infection or inflammation in a meibomian gland (of the eyelid). If chronic, it is called a chalazion.

HOTV. Test chart that uses these four letters for assessing vision in pre-school children. Responses consist of matching an identified letter with the same letter on a card.

hyaloid canal. See CLOQUET'S CANAL.

hyperopia (hi-pur-OH-pee-uh), **farsightedness, hypermetropia.** Focusing defect in which an eye is underpowered. Thus light rays coming from a distant object strike the retina before coming to sharp focus; true focus is said to be "behind the retina." Corrected with additional optical power, which may be supplied by a plus lens (spectacle or contact) or by excessive use of the eye's own focusing ability (accommodation).

hyperphoria (H) (hi-pur-FOR-ee-uh). Tendency toward upward deviation that occurs only when the eye is covered; when uncovered, the eye straightens.

hypertropia (HT) (hi-pur-TROH-pee-uh). Upward deviation of one eye while other remains straight and fixates normally.

hyphema (hi-FEE-muh). Blood in the anterior chamber, such as following blunt trauma to the eyeball.

hypopyon (hi-POH-pee-un). Accumulation of pus in the anterior chamber.

hypotropia (hi-poh-TROH-pee-uh). Downward deviation of one eye while other remains straight and fixates normally.

I

induced tropia test (ITT). For detection of fixation preference in aligned eyes; a prism is used (10^Δ vertically or 25^Δ horizontally) to induce a misalignment in corneal reflex position.

infantile esotropia. See ESOTROPIA.

infantile glaucoma. See GLAUCOMA.

inferior oblique (IO) (oh-BLEEK or oh-BLIKE). Extraocular muscle attached to the lower, outer side of the eyeball behind the equator. Three functions: extorsion (rotating top of eye away from nose, especially on outward movement), elevation (especially on inward movement); and abduction (outward eye movement). Innervated by the 3rd (oculomotor) cranial nerve.

inferior rectus (IR). Extraocular muscle attached to underside of the eyeball (globe). Three functions: depression (moves eye downward, especially when it is turned out); extorsion (rotates eye outward, especially on inward gaze), and adduction (inward eye movement). Innervated by the 3rd (oculomotor) cranial nerve.

iridocyclitis. See UVEITIS.

intermittent strabismus (struh-BIZ-mis). See STRABISMUS.

iritis (i-RI-tis). Inflammation of the iris. Can cause pain, tearing, blurred vision, small pupil (miosis) and a red congested eye.

J K L

jaw winking syndrome, external pterygoid-levator synkinesis, Marcus Gunn jaw winking syndrome. Droopy eyelid (ptosis) that opens wide upon chewing, sucking, or moving the mouth to the opposite side. Caused by abnormal innervation of the levator muscle by the 5th (trigeminal) cranial nerve.

keratitis (KEHR-uh-TI-tis). Corneal inflammation, characterized by loss of luster and transparency, and cellular infiltration.

keratoconjunctivitis (KEHR-uh-toh-kun junk-tih-VI-tis). Inflammation involving both the cornea and conjunctiva.

keratoconus (kehr-uh-toh-KOH-nus). Degenerative corneal disease affecting vision. Characterized by generalized thinning and cone-shaped protrusion of the central cornea, usually in both eyes. Becomes apparent during 2nd decade of life. Hereditary.

keratoplasty (KEHR-uh-toh-plas-tee). See CORNEAL TRANSPLANT.

Kestenbaum procedure. Method of strengthening or weakening both medial rectus and lateral rectus muscles, so an individual with nystagmus (side-to-side eye movements) will not need to hold head in an abnormal position to see well. The position with least eye movement (null point) is repositioned straight ahead.

Knapp procedure. Transposition of lateral and medial rectus muscles to either side of the superior rectus to correct a downward eye deviation (hypotropia).

KPs (keratic precipitates). Inflammatory cells and white blood cells from the iris and ciliary body that enter the aqueous and adhere to the innermost corneal surface (endothelium). Called "mutton fat" if KPs are large clusters (granulomatous) or "punctate" if smaller (nongranulomatous). Typical finding in various types of uveitis.

Krimsky method. Assessment of eye deviation by using prisms to equalize the position of the corneal light reflex within each pupil.

lacrimal apparatus (LAK-rih-mul), **tear drainage system**. Orbital structures for tear production and drainage. Tears (produced in lacrimal gland above eyeball) flow across the corneal surface, drain into the upper and lower puncta (openings at inner eyelid margins), through the upper and lower canaliculi to the common canaliculus, into the tear sac, then through the nasolacrimal duct into the nose.

lacrimal canaliculus. See CANALICULUS.

lacrimal duct. See TEAR DUCT.

lacrimal gland. Almond-shaped structure that produces tears. Located at upper outer region of orbit, above the eyeball.

lacrimal lake. Pool of tears in lower conjunctival cul-de-sac that drains into the openings (puncta) of tear drainage system.

lacrimal probe. Thin rod used for clearing obstructions in the tear drainage system.

lacrimal sac. See TEAR SAC.

lateral rectus palsy. See ABDUCENS PALSY.

lazy eye. See AMBLYOPIA.

Leber's congenital amaurosis. See CONGENITAL AMAUROSIS.

lensectomy. Removal of a lens.

leukocoria (lu-koh-KOR-ee-uh). Any eye condition that whitens the pupil.

lens capsule. See CAPSULE.

levator resection (luh-VAY-tur). Repair of a drooping eyelid (ptosis) by shortening the levator muscle in the upper lid.

M

macula, macula lutea (LU-tee-uh). Literally, "yellow spot." Small (3°) central area of the retina surrounding the fovea; area of acute central vision.

major amblyoscope (AM-blee-uh-skohp). Binocular viewing system that permits simultaneous presentation of separate fixation targets (usually on slides) for each eye. Used in evaluation and treatment of strabismus and other binocularity problems.

Marcus Gunn jaw winking syndrome. See JAW WINKING SYNDROME.

Marcus-Gunn pupil (MG), Gunn pupil, afferent (or) **relative afferent pupillary defect**. Diminished pupil reaction to light, usually secondary to optic nerve disease that causes slowed conduction in optic nerve fibers. In dim illumination, a sudden bright light stimulus to the normal eye will result in both pupils contracting briskly. When the light stimulus is shifted to the defective eye, the pupils contract less well, so they appear to enlarge.

medial rectus (MR). Extraocular muscle that moves the eye inward from the straight-ahead position (adduction). Attached to the outside of the eyeball on the nasal side. Innervated by the 3rd (oculomotor) cranial nerve.

meibomian gland (mi-BOH-mee-un), **tarsal gland**. Oil gland (one of a series) within eyelid tissue (tarsus) whose duct opens onto the eyelid margin just behind the gray line. Secretions supply the outer portion of tear film, preventing rapid tear evaporation and tear overflow and providing tight eyelid closure.

mesodermal dysgenesis of cornea. See ANTERIOR CHAMBER CLEAVAGE SYNDROME.

mesodermal dysgenesis of iris. See RIEGER'S SYNDROME.

microphthalmia (mi-krahf-THAL-mee-uh), **microphthalmos**. Abnormally small eyeball.

micropsia (mi-KRAHP-see-uh). Disturbance of visual perception in which objects appear smaller than true size.

microstrabismus (mi-kroh-struh-BIZ-mus), **microtropia, monofixation syndrome, small angle strabismus**. Eye misalignment with a small, usually inward, deviation and some fusion ability. Deviation usually increases with disruption of fusion (as with covering one eye). Affected eye may be amblyopic and/or anisometropic, usually with a small central suppression scotoma.

Möbius' (*or* Moebius) syndrome (MEE-bee-us or MOH-bee-us), **congenital bulbar paralysis** *(or)* **facial diplegia, von Graefe's syndrome**. Bilateral malformation in the cranial nuclei of the 6th (abducens) and 7th (facial) nerves. Results in inability to move either eye outward past the midline or close the eyelids, a large inward eye deviation (esotropia), and an expressionless facial appearance.

monochromacy. See ACHROMATOPSIA.

monofixation syndrome. See MICROSTRABISMUS.

motility (ocular). See OCULAR MOTILITY.

mydriatic (mid-ree-AT-ik). Drug that stimulates sympathetic nerve fibers, causing the iris dilator to contract (dilating the pupils), or blocking parasympathetic nerve fibers (paralyzing the iris sphincter muscle). Examples: Atropine, Cyclogyl, Mydriacyl, Neosynephrine.

myopexy (retroequatorial). See RETROEQUATORIAL MYOPEXY.

myopia (mi-OH-pee-uh), **nearsightedness**. Focusing defect in which eye is overpowered. Light rays coming from a distant object are brought to focus in front of the retina. Requires a minus lens correction to "weaken" the eye optically and permit clear distance vision.

N

nasolacrimal duct. See TEAR DUCT.

nasolacrimal duct obstruction. See BLOCKED TEAR DUCT.

nasolacrimal probing. See PROBING.

night blindness, nyctalopia. Inefficient dark adaptation that results in markedly reduced vision in dim light. Usually indicates a defect in the (retinal) rods. May be progressive.

noncomitant strabismus. See STRABISMUS.

null point. Position of gaze where eye movements of congenital nystagmus are reduced or eliminated.

nyctalopia (nik-tuh-LOH-pee-uh). See NIGHT BLINDNESS.

nystagmus (ni-STAG-mus). Involuntary, rhythmic side-to-side or up and down (oscillating) eye movements that are faster in one direction than the other.

    congenital: noted within first 6 months of life. There is usually one position of gaze in which the spontaneous movements are minimized or absent (null point). May be hereditary or result from decreased vision from corneal opacities, cataracts, albinism, chorioretinitis, aniridia, macular disease, or optic atrophy.

O

occlusion amblyopia (am-blee-OH-pee-uh). See AMBLYOPIA.

ocular albinism (AL-bin-iz-um). Lack of pigment (may be partial) in the iris and choroid. Results in reddish pupils and iris (from choroidal vessels seen through overlying retina). Usually accompanied by poor vision, light sensitivity (photophobia), involuntary oscillating eye movements (nystagmus).

ocular motility, motility. Deals with extraocular muscles and their effect on eye movements. .

ocular torticollis (tor-tih-KOL-is). Abnormal head turn or tilt that develops to compensate for asymetric nystagmus or incomitant strabismus.

Oculinum (ahk-yu-LI-num). Trade name for botulinum toxin; used as an alternative or in addition to surgery to correct eye misalignments.

oculo-digital reflex. Constant rubbing or pressing on the eyes with the fists or fingers. Common in blind children.

oculomotor apraxia (ay-PRAKS-ee-uh). See CONGENITAL OCULOMOTOR APRAXIA.

ophthalmia neonatorum (ahf-THAL-mee-uh nee-oh-nuh-TOR-um). Severe eye infection of newborn infants acquired in the birth canal.

ophthalmoscope (ahf-THAL-muh-skohp). Illuminated instrument for visualizing the interior of the eye (especially the fundus).

    direct: provides a magnified (15x) upright view with a small (8°) field of view; consists of a bright light source and incorporated focusing lenses.

    indirect: creates an inverted, magnified (3x) image of the fundus projected in front of the eye, with a wide (30°) field of view. Consists of a bright light source and hand-held high-plus lens. Binocular model allows stereoscopic depth perception of the fundus.

optic chiasm. See CHIASM.

optic cup. 1. White depression in center of optic disc; usually occupies 1/3 or less of the total disc diameter. 2. Early stage in a developing eye; outpouching from the primitive brain.

optic disc, disc, optic nerve head. Ocular end of the optic nerve. Denotes the exit of retinal nerve fibers from the eye and entrance of blood vessels to the eye.

optic nerve. Second cranial nerve. Largest sensory nerve of the eye; carries impulses for sight from the retina to the brain. Composed of retinal nerve fibers that exit the eyeball through the optic disc and exit the orbit through the optic foramen.

optic nerve head. See OPTIC DISC.

optic nerve hypoplasia (hi-poh-PLAY-zhuh). Congenitally small optic disc; sometimes surrounded by a double ring (scleral halo) and often a pigment epithelium halo. Vision may or may not be reduced.

orbit. Pyramid-shaped cavity in the skull (apex toward back of head), about 2 inches deep and lined by the orbital bones (ethmoid, frontal, lacrimal, maxillary, nasal, palatine, sphenoid). Contains the eyeball, its muscles, blood supply, nerve supply and fat.

orthoptics. Discipline dealing with the diagnosis and treatment of defective eye coordination, binocular vision, and functional amblyopia by non-medical and non-surgical methods, e.g., glasses, prisms, exercises.

orthoptist (or-THAHP-tist). Certified allied health person in ophthalmology who analyzes and treats patients with dysfunctions of binocularity and/or ocular motility.

oscillopsia (ahs-sil-AHP-see-uh). Illusion of object movement; accompanies acquired nystagmus.

P

papilledema (pap-il-uh-DEE-muh), **choked disc.** Swelling of the optic disc with engorged blood vessels, associated with elevated pressure within the skull. Characterized by blurred optic disc edges, flame-shaped nerve fiber layer hemorrhages next to the disc, and an enlarged physiologic blind spot. Vision is normal.

paradoxic pupil. Any unexpected pupillary reaction, e.g., when pupil is expected to contract with light stimulation, it dilates, and vice versa. Seen with optic nerve hypoplasia, achromatopsia, congenital stationary night blindness.

patching. Covering an amblyopic patient's preferred eye by occlusion, to improve vision in the other eye.

penalization (peh-nul-ih-ZAY-shun). Treatment of amblyopia with atropine, miotics or special glasses, to handicap one eye in order to force the use of the amblyopic eye.

perimetry (puh-RIM-ih-tree). Method of charting extent of a stationary eye's field of vision with test objects of various sizes and light intensities. Aids in detection of damage to sensory visual pathways.

Peter anomaly. See ANTERIOR CHAMBER CLEAVAGE SYNDROME.

phoria (FOR-ee-uh), **heterophoria**. Latent tendency of eyes to deviate that is prevented by fusion. Thus a deviation occurs only when a cover is placed over an eye; when uncovered, the eye straightens.

phoropter (FOR-ahp-tur, for-AHP-tur). Refraction device for determining an eye's optical correction. Incorporates spherical and cylindrical lenses, prisms, occluders and pinholes.

photophobia (foh-toh-FOH-bee-uh). Abnormal sensitivity to, and discomfort from, light; may be associated with excessive tearing. Often due to inflammation of the iris or cornea.

PHPV (persistent hyperplasia of the primary vitreous, persistent hyperplastic primary vitreous). Congenital anomaly: embryologic malformation caused by failure of normal regression of primary vitreous and hyaloid vascular system. Affected eye is usually slightly small (microphthalmic) with elongated ciliary processes, a shallow anterior chamber, cataract, and a white fibrovascular tract extending from the disc into the vitreous.

phthisis bulbi (TI-sis BUL-bi), **phthisical eye**. Diseased or damaged eyeball that has lost function and shrunk. Associated with low intraocular pressure because the ciliary body stops producing aqueous fluid.

pigment epithelium. See RETINAL PIGMENT EPITHELIUM.

pinguecula (pin-GWEK-yu-luh). Yellowish-brown subconjunctival elevation composed of degenerated elastic tissue; may occur on either side of the cornea. Benign. Plural: pingueculae.

pink eye. See CONJUNCTIVITIS.

posterior fixation suture. See RETROEQUATORIAL MYOPEXY.

posterior segment. Rear two-thirds of eyeball (behind the lens); includes the vitreous, retina, optic disc, choroid, pars plana, and most of the sclera.

presbyopia (prez-bee-OH-pee-uh). Refractive condition in which there is a diminished power of accommodation arising from loss of elasticity of the crystalline lens, as occurs with aging. Usually becomes significant after age 45.

pre-septal cellulitis. See CELLULITIS.

primary deviation. Amount of eye deviation caused by a paralyzed muscle, measured when the normal eye is fixating.

primary open angle glaucoma (POAG). See GLAUCOMA.

prism. See BASE-DOWN BASE-IN, BASE-OUT or BASE-UP PRISM.

prism adaptation test (PAT). Fresnel prisms are placed over eyeglass lenses in an attempt to gain binocular control of an eye misalignment.

prism + alternate cover test. See COVER TEST.

prism diopter (di-AHP-tur) (Δ). 1. Prism strength: 1^Δ indicates deflection of a light ray by 1 cm at a distance of 1 m. 2. 1 arc degree of eye deviation = 1.7^Δ (approx.).

probing, nasolacrimal probing. Opening tear drainage system by passing a thin rod through the passageway and pressing gently to break any obstruction.

prosthesis. See SHELL.

pseudophakia (SU-doh-FAY-kee-uh). State of an intraocular lens implant taking the place of the eye's natural lens.

pterygium (tur-IH-jee-um). Abnormal wedge-shaped growth on the bulbar conjunctiva. May gradually advance onto the cornea and require surgical removal. Probably related to sun irritation. Plural: pterygia.

ptosis (TOH-sis), **blepharoptosis**. Drooping of upper eyelid. May be congenital or caused by paralysis or weakness (paresis) of the 3rd (oculomotor) cranial nerve or sympathetic nerves, or by excessive weight of the upper lids.

punctate keratitis (kehr-uh-TI-tus), **superficial** (or) **Thygeson's superficial punctate keratitis**. Corneal disease of unknown cause, characterized by small superficial corneal lesions. Other symptoms include foreign body sensation and sensitivity to bright light. Sometimes recurs after spontaneous remissions.

punctum (PUNK-tum). Tiny skin opening of the lacrimal canaliculus of each upper and lower eyelid, near the nose. Entrance to the tear drainage (lacrimal) system. Plural: puncta.

    inferior: opening in the papilla (elevation) of the lower eyelid margin). Lower entrance to the tear drainage system. Also called lower punctum.

    superior: opening in the papilla (elevation) of the upper eyelid margin. Upper entrance to the eye's tear drainage system. Also called upper punctum.

pupillotonia. See ADIE'S PUPIL.

R

recession. Weakening an overactive extraocular muscle to correct an eye deviation. Muscle is removed from its insertion and repositioned farther back on the eyeball (globe).

recess-resect (R & R). For correcting an eye deviation; one extraocular muscle is repositioned farther back on eyeball to weaken it and its opposing muscle in the same eye (direct antagonist) is shortened, to strengthen it.

red reflex. Normal red glow emerging from the pupil when the interior of the eye is illuminated.

reflex. 1. Involuntary response to a stimulus. 2. Slang for reflection.

    corneal: 1. Neurologic response: blink caused by touching the cornea. 2. Mirror-like reflection of a bright light from the corneal surface.

    oculo-cardiac: decrease in heart rate following manipulation of the eyes or extraocular muscles.

    oculo-cephalic (sef-AL-ik): involuntary eye rotation in the opposite direction from head rotation to maintain fixation on a non-moving target. May be abnormal with some brainstem defects.

    oculo-digital: constant rubbing or pressing on the eyes with the fists or fingers; common in blind children.

    pupillary: decrease in pupil size (constriction) that occurs with direct light stimulation to eye.

    vestibulo-ocular: same as OCULO-CEPHALIC (above).

refraction. 1. Bending of light rays as they travel from a clear medium to another of different density. 2. Determination of an eye's refractive error and the best corrective lenses to be prescribed; series of lenses in graded powers are presented to determine which provide sharpest, clearest vision. 3. Prescription for eyeglasses or contact lenses resulting from this test.

    cycloplegic: test performed after lens accommodation has been paralyzed with cycloplegic eyedrops. Eliminates variability in optical power caused by a contracting lens.

    manifest: test performed without cycloplegic eyedrops.

refractive error. Optical defect in an unaccommodating eye; parallel light rays are not brought to a sharp focus precisely on the retina, producing a blurred retinal image. Can be corrected by eyeglasses or contact lenses.

refractive surgery, keratorefractive surgery. Various procedures that alter the shape of the cornea and thus how it bends light, in order to change the eye's refractive error (arcuate keratotomy, epikeratophakia, keratomileusis, keratophakia, laser sculpting, LASIK, photorefractive surgery, radial keratotomy, refractive keratoplasty, thermoplasty, transverse keratotomy).

relative afferent pupillary defect (RAPD) (AF-ur-unt). See Marcus-Gunn pupil.

retina (RET-ih-nuh), **tunica nervosa oculi**. Part of the eye (embryologically part of brain) that converts images from the eye's optical system into electrical impulses that are sent along the optic nerve for transmission to the brain. Forms a thin membranous lining of the rear two-thirds of the globe. Consists of layers that include rods and cones; bipolar, amacrine, ganglion, horizontal and Müller cells; and all interconnecting nerve fibers.

retinal correspondence. Inherent relationship between paired retinal visual cells in the two eyes. Images from an object stimulate both cells, which transmit the information to the brain, permitting a single visual impression localized in the same direction in space.

    abnormal: same as anomalous (below).

    anomalous: binocular sensory adaptation to compensate for a long- standing eye deviation; fovea of the straight (non-deviated) eye and a non- foveal retinal point of the deviated eye work together, sometimes permitting single binocular vision despite the misalignment.

    normal: both foveae work together as corresponding retinal points, with resultant images blended (fused) in the occipital cortex of the brain.

retinal detachment (RD), retinal separation. Separation of sensory retina from the underlying pigment epithelium. Disrupts visual cell structure and thus markedly disturbs vision. Almost always caused by a retinal tear; often requires immediate surgical repair.

retinal pigment epithelium (RPE) (ep-ih-THEE-lee-um), **pigment epithelium**. Pigment cell layer (hexagonal cells densely packed with pigment granules) just outside the retina that nourishes retinal visual cells. Firmly attached to underlying choroid and overlying retinal visual cells.

retinitis pigmentosa. Progressive retinal degeneration in both eyes. Night blindness, usually in childhood, is followed by loss of peripheral vision (initially as a ring-shaped defect), progressing over many years to tunnel vision and finally blindness. Hereditary.

retinoblastoma (ret-in-noh-blas-TOH-muh). Malignant intraocular tumor that develops from retinal visual cells. If untreated, seedling nodules produce secondary tumors that gradually fill the eye and extend along the optic nerve to the brain, ending in death. Most common childhood ocular malignancy. Hereditary.

retinopathy of prematurity (ROP). Series of destructive retinal changes that may develop in premature infants. In the active stage, findings include dilated, tortuous peripheral blood vessels, retinal hemorrhages and abnormal newly formed blood vessels (neovascularization). Sometimes regresses; other times a peripheral fibrotic scar forms that detaches the retina. Can result in vision loss or blindness. Other possible complications: glaucoma, cataracts, myopia (nearsightedness), sunken eyes, and eye misalignment. Previously called retrolental fibroplasia.

retinoscope (RET-in-oh-skohp). Hand-held device for measuring an eye's refractive error with no response required from the patient. Light is projected into the eye, and the movements of the light reflection from the eye are neutralized (eliminated) with lenses.

retroequatorial myopexy (RET-roh-ee-kwuh-TOR-ee-ul MI-oh-pek-see), **Faden procedure, posterior fixation suture**. Method of weakening a rectus muscle (medial, lateral, superior or inferior) by suturing it to the sclera 10–16 mm behind its insertion, restricting its action.

rhabdomyosarcoma (RAB-doh-mi-oh-sahr-KOH-muh). Highly malignant tumor of striated muscle in children; can affect orbital area.

Rieger syndrome (REE-gurz), **mesodermal dysgenesis of iris**. Genetic defect occurring in the 5th or 6th week of fetal development. Eye findings include glaucoma, underdeveloped iris, deformed pupil, prominent Schwalbe's ring, corneal defects, and astigmatism.

rigid gas permeable lens (RGP), gas permeable lens. Rigid plastic contact lens that allows oxygen and carbon dioxide penetration.

rod monochromacy. Rare congenital inability to distinguish colors as a result of absent or nonfunctioning retinal cones. Associated with light sensitivity (photophobia), involuntary eye oscillations (nystagmus) and poor vision. Nonprogressive.

S

Schlemm's canal (shlemz). Circular channel deep in corneoscleral junction (limbus) that carries aqueous fluid from the anterior chamber of the eye to the bloodstream.

sclera (SKLEH-ruh). Opaque, fibrous, protective outer layer of the eye ("white of the eye") that is directly continuous with the cornea in front and with the sheath covering the optic nerve behind. Contains collagen and elastic fibers. Plural: sclerae.

secondary cataract, after-cataract. Remnants of the opaque lens remaining in the eye or opacities forming after extracapsular cataract removal.

secondary deviation. Amount of deviation measured when an eye with a weak or restricted extraocular muscle fixates. Greater than a primary deviation.

secondary implant. Intraocular lens implanted into an eye (to replace an extracted cataract), done as a second surgical procedure at a later date than the original surgery.

"setting sun" phenomenon. Down-gaze eye position with upper eyelid retraction, exposing the upper white part of the eye (sclera); creates a staring expression. May be associated with congenital hydrocephalus.

shallow angle. Shallower-than-normal space between the iris and cornea. Increases potential for restricting drainage of aqueous fluid through the trabecular meshwork.

shell, prosthesis. Cosmetic "false eye" replacement for a removed (enucleated) eye. Plexiglas shell painted to resemble a natural eye fits into the conjunctival sac under the eyelids and over a buried implant.

silicone lens. Oxygen-permeable contact lens that is soft, flexible, and maintains its size and shape whether or not it is kept in a solution.

sixth nerve palsy. See ABDUCENS PALSY.

simultaneous prism and cover test (SPCT). See COVER TEST.

small angle strabismus. See MICROSTRABISMUS.

Snellen chart. Test chart for assessing visual acuity. Contains rows of letters, numbers, or symbols in standardized graded sizes, with designated distance at which each row should be legible to a normal eye. Usually tested at 6 m (20 ft.).

soft contact lens (SCL). Water-absorbing (hydrophilic) small plastic disc used for correcting refractive error or protecting a damaged corneal surface. Rests on cornea; often more comfortable and easier to tolerate than a hard contact lens.

spasmus nutans (SPAZ-mus NU-tanz). Fine, rapid eye oscillations (nystagmus) and head nodding, often with a head tilt. Appears in 1st or 2nd year of life, then gradually subsides. Usually harmless, but may herald brainstesm tumor.

Stargardt's disease (STAHR-gahrtz). Macular degeneration characterized by central vision loss with minimal ophthalmoscopic changes. Later, the macula may show pigment clumping surrounded by a hammered-metal appearance. Occurs between ages 6–20. Hereditary.

stereopsis (stehr-ee-AHP-sis). See BINOCULAR DEPTH PERCEPTION.

strabismic amblyopia. See AMBLYOPIA.

strabismus (struh-BIZ-mus), **deviation, heterotropia, squint, tropia**. Eye misalignment caused by extraocular muscle imbalance: one fovea is not directed at the same object as the other. Present even when both eyes uncovered.

    alternating: continuous changing between a deviating right eye and straight left eye, and a deviating left eye and straight right eye.

    antipodean: one eye turns in; when it straightens, the other eye turns out.

    comitant, concomitant: the amount of deviation remains the same in every direction of gaze.

    horizontal: one eye deviates inward or outward.

    incomitant: degree of misalignment changes in different positions of gaze because an extraocular muscle is paretic, paralytic or restricted.

    intermittent: any eye deviation in which eyes are sometimes straight, and other times one eye is straight and the other deviates.

    noncomitant. same as INCOMITANT (above).

    primary: (smaller) deviation caused by a paralyzed muscle when the uninvolved eye is fixating.

    secondary: (larger) deviation caused by a paralyzed muscle when the involved eye is fixating.

    small angle. See MICROSTRABISMUS.

    vertical: one eye is higher or lower than the other.

strabismus fixus. Congenital defect: eye(s) are fixed in an extreme position due to tightened medial or lateral recti muscles. Results in the eyes deviating either inward (esotropia) or outward (exotropia).

stye. See HORDEOLUM.

superior oblique palsy. See FOURTH NERVE PALSY.

superior oblique tendon sheath syndrome, Brown's (or) sheath syndrome. Sheath of superior oblique muscle that does not, or cannot, relax when the eye attempts to look upward and inward; mimics an inferior oblique palsy. Unilateral; may be congenital or acquired.

suppression. Subconscious inhibition of an eye's retinal image. Usually occurs in strabismus when a deviated eye's image interferes with that received from the straight eye. Unconscious mechanism to avoid double vision (diplopia).

symblepharon (sim-BLEF-uh-rahn). Abnormal adhesion of eyelid (palpebral) conjunctiva to eyeball (bulbar) conjunctiva.

synechia (sin-EEK-ee-uh). Adhesion(s) that bind the iris to any adjacent structures. Plural: synechiae.

    anterior: between the iris and the cornea.

    peripheral anterior: between the iris periphery and the cornea. Occurs with unrelieved attacks of angle-closure glaucoma; may occur following injury or surgery.

    posterior: between the iris and the lens. Occurs commonly in uveitis.

T

tarsal gland (TAR-sul). See MEIBOMIAN GLAND.

tarsorrhaphy (tar-SOR-uh-fee). Stitching upper and lower eyelids together, partially or completely, usually to provide temporary protection to the eye. Plural: tarsorrhaphies.

tarsus (TAHR-sus), **tarsal plate**. Dense plate-like framework within the upper and lower eyelids that provides stiffness and shape. Plural: tarsi.

tear drainage system. See LACRIMAL APPARATUS.

tear duct, lacrimal (or) nasolacrimal duct. Tear drainage channel that extends from the lacrimal sac to an opening in the mucous membrane of the nose.

tear sac, lacrimal sac. Tear collecting structure lying under the skin near the bridge of the nose. Tears enter from the common canaliculus and leave from the lacrimal duct into the nose.

Teller acuity cards (TAC). Measures visual acuity in young non-verbal children by testing their ability to detect alternating black and white stripes of varying widths (spatial frequencies).

Tenon's capsule, fascia bulbi. Thin, fibrous, somewhat elastic membrane that envelops the eyeball from the limbus (edge of the cornea) to the optic nerve; attaches loosely to the sclera and to extraocular muscle tendons.

tenotomy (ten-AH-tuh-mee). Cutting a tendon without actually removing any severed tissue. Weakens action of the muscle to which it is attached.

thyroid eye disease. See GRAVES' DISEASE.

third nerve (N III) palsy. Weakness of the muscles innervated by the 3rd (oculomotor) cranial nerve: includes the eyelid levator, inferior oblique, medial rectus, inferior rectus and superior rectus muscles, and sometimes the pupillary sphincter and ciliary muscles. The involved eye usually deviates outward and slightly downward and has an extremely droopy (ptotic) upper eyelid without its lid fold; sometimes the pupil is dilated and accommodation is reduced.

tonic pupil. See ADIE'S PUPIL.

tonometer. See APPLANATION TONOMETER.

torticollis (ocular). See OCULAR TORTICOLLIS.

traction test. See FORCED DUCTION TEST.

transillumination. Use of an intense light beam (e.g., slit lamp or small flashlight) to shine through translucent eye tissue to better visualize ocular tumors, cysts or hemorrhages in sillhouette.

trichiasis (trih-KI-uh-sus). Misdirected upper or lower eyelashes that turn inward toward the eyeball; may scratch the cornea. Usually follows severe eyelid inflammation or scarring.

trochlea (TROH-klee-uh). Ring-like cartilage attached nasally to the frontal bone along the upper orbital rim. Acts as a pulley for the tendon of the superior oblique muscle.

trochlear nerve (TROH-klee-ur). Fourth cranial nerve. Motor nerve that innervates the superior oblique muscle of the eye. Originates in the lower midbrain; enters the orbit through the superior orbital fissure.

tropia (TROH-pee-uh). See STRABISMUS.

tunica vasculosa lentis (vas-kyu-LOH-suh LEN-tis). Embryonic blood vessel network covering the back of the lens until the 5th month of fetal life.

Tyndall effect. SEE AQUEOUS FLARE.

U V Z

ulcer (corneal). Area of epithelial tissue loss from the corneal surface; associated with inflammatory cells in the cornea and anterior chamber. Usually caused by a bacterial, fungal or viral infection.

uvea (YU-vee-uh), **uveal tract**. Pigmented layers of the eye (iris, ciliary body, choroid) that contain most of the intraocular blood vessels.

uveitis (yu-vee-I-tis). Inflammation of any of the structures of the uvea: iris, ciliary body, or choroid. Plural: uveitides.

    anterior: inflammation of iris or ciliary body. Also called iridocyclitis.

    endogenous: thought to arise from causes within the body.

    posterior: inflammation of the choroid.

vergence ability, amplitudes, fusional amplitudes. Amount (in diopters) the eyes can move inward (converge) added to the amount they can move outward (diverge), while maintaining single vision.

vernal conjunctivitis, vernal catarrh. Allergic conjunctival inflammation, with itching and excess mucous, recurring in children during warm weather. Numerous small lumps (papillae) form on the palpebral conjunctiva. Scrapings exhibit many eosinophils.

version. See CONJUGATE MOVEMENT.

visual acuity. Assessment of the eye's ability to distinguish object details and shapes, using the smallest identifiable object that can be seen at a specified distance (usually 20 ft. or 16 in.).

visual axis, line of fixation, primary line of sight, principal line of direction, visual line. Imaginary line connecting a viewed object and the fovea.

visual cortex (primary), Brodmann area 17, striate area. Area (cerebral end of sensory visual pathways) in the occipital lobes of the brain, where initial conscious registration of visual information takes place.

visual evoked response (VER), visual evoked cortical potential. Computerized recording of electrical activity in the occipital cortex (back of brain) that results from stimulating the retina with light flashes. Used for detecting defects in the retina-to-brain nerve pathway (which can change brain wave patterns).

visual field, field of vision. Full extent of the area visible to an eye that is fixating straight ahead. Measured in degrees from fixation.

vitreous (VIT-ree-us), **vitreous body** (or) **gel** (or) **humor**. Transparent, colorless gelatinous mass (fine collagen fibrils and hyaluronic acid) that fills the rear two-thirds of the eyeball, between the lens and the retina.

V pattern. Horizontal eye misalignment in which an inturning (esotropic) eye deviates more on down-gaze than than on up-gaze, or an outward turning (exotropic) eye deviates more on up-gaze than on down-gaze.

wall-eyes. See EXOTROPIA.

zonules (ZAHN-yoolz), Radially arranged fibers that suspend the lens from the ciliary body and hold it in position.

Suggested Reading

Brodsky MC, Baker RS, Hamed LM. *Pediatric Neuro-ophthalmolony*. New York: Springer Verlag; 1995.

Calhoun JH, Nelson LB, Harley RD. *Atlas of Pediatric Ophthalmology Surgery*. Philadelphia: Saunders; 1987.

Del Monte MA. *Atlas of Pediatric Ophthalmology and Strabismus Surgery*. New York: Churchill Livingstone; 1993.

Helveston EM. *Surgical Management of Strabismus: An Atlas of Strabismus Surgery*. 4th ed. St. Louis: Mosby; 1993.

Helveston EM, Ellis FD. *Pediatric Ophthalmology Practice*. 2nd ed. St. Louis: Mosby; 1984.

Nelson LB, Calhoun JH, Harley RD. *Pediatric Ophthalmology*. 3rd ed. Philadelphia: Saunders; 1991.

Pratt-Johnson JA, Tillson G. *Management of Strabismus and Amblyopia: A Practical Guide*. New York: Thieme; 1994.

Tasman W, Jaeger EA, eds. *Duane's Clinical Ophthalmology*. Philadelphia: Lippincott-Raven; 1996.

Taylor D. *Pediatric Ophthalmology*. 2nd ed. Cambridge, MA: Blackwell Science; 1997.

Von Noorden GK. *Binocular Vision and Ocular Motility: Theory and Management of Strabismus*. 5th ed. St. Louis: Mosby; 1996.

Wright KW, ed. *Pediatric Ophthalmology and Strabismus*. St. Louis: Mosby; 1995.

Index

Additional copies of *A Child's Eyes* are available from the publisher at $39.95 each plus shipping/handling of $8.00 per order.

Credit card orders and requests for information may be faxed to
1-800-854-4947

Or write:
Triad Publishing Company
P.O. Box 13355
Gainesville, FL 32604

Books and software of related interest:

• *Dictionary of Eye Terminology*, 3rd ed., by Barbara Cassin and Sheila Solomon. Melvin Rubin, MD, editor. Over 5,000 of the most frequently used terms, phrases and abbreviations associated with the eye and vision. Written in "plain English."

• *EyeCheck* — ophthalmic word spell-checker of over 20,000 terms: medical, technical and scientific words, trade and generic drug names, and more. Once installed, it becomes part of the regular spell checker in your word processing program.
For PC (Word, any version; Word Perfect, version 5.0, 5.1, 6.0, 6.1) or Mac (Word 5.0, 5.1).

• *Triad's Eye Care Notes*, by Lawrence Winograd, MD and Melvin L. Rubin, MD, with a panel of contributors. Patient education handouts of over 100 eye diseases and conditions, explained simply and accurately as though you were talking to your patient.
Annual revisions and new topics. Text (looseleaf pages to photocopy) and software (Windows) formats.